MW01069176

The
Graded Motor Imagery
Handbook

G. Lorimer Moseley
David S. Butler
Timothy B. Beames
Thomas J. Giles

Cover artwork and illustration
Dan Tomkins

Noigroup Publications
Adelaide, Australia, 2012
www.noigroup.com
www.gradedmotorimagery.com
www.noigroup.com/recognise

Published by Noigroup Publications for NOI Australasia, Pty Ltd.

Printed and bound by van Gastel TPM, Adelaide, Australia.

The procedures and practices described in this book should be implemented in a manner consistent with professional standards set for the circumstances that apply in each situation. Every effort has been made to confirm accuracy of the information presented and to correctly relate generally accepted practices.

The authors, editor and publisher cannot accept responsibility for errors or exclusions or for the outcome of the application of the material presented herein. There is no expressed or implied warranty of this book or information imparted by it.

National Library of Australia
A catalogue record for this book is available from the National Library of Australia

State Library of South Australia
A catalogue record for this book is available from the State Library of South Australia.

Moseley, G. Lorimer, Butler, David S.,
Beames, Timothy B., Giles, Thomas J.
The Graded Motor Imagery Handbook
First edition March 2012, reprint August 2012
Includes index

ISBN 978-0-9872467-5-2

Noigroup Publications
NOI Australasia Pty Ltd
19 North Street, Adelaide City West,
South Australia 5000
www.noigroup.com
Telephone +61 (0)8 8211 6388
Facsimile +61 (0)8 8211 8909
info@noigroup.com

MIX
Paper from
responsible sources
FSC® C018479

Acknowledgements

We would like to thank the production team at NOI HQ – the design team Paula Filippone and Ariane Allchurch, editor Juliet Gore, research Kat Waterman, accounts Karin Kosiol, dispatch and customer service Tara Gagliardi, as well as Dan Tomkins for his great artwork and Halton Stewart for his ongoing enthusiasm and innovation in developing computer-based tools.

But mostly, we want to thank the very large number of patients who tried out various forms of GMI during its development, or who participated in experiments and clinical trials on it once it was developed and the community of clinicians who continually feed back their experiences of GMI in the real world so that we can keep working towards better outcomes for people in pain.

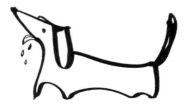

Contents

Knowledge
– The power behind
Graded Motor Imagery
David S. Butler

1. INTRODUCTION

I'm a physiotherapist by trade and ever since I graduated back in 1978, I have encountered a group of patients who have defied any therapeutic attempts – be they surgical, pharmacological or any of the numerous strategies that the rehabilitation world offers. And as if to taunt me they would say things like 'my arm doesn't feel like mine' or 'it hurts when I think of moving' or the pain would move around their body and you could never catch it. Vagueness was a symptom in itself and it was difficult to see past my frustration to what lay behind the patient's vagueness. I am glad I am still a physio, still involved in rehabilitation because I believe I have just caught a new era in rehabilitation science – a refreshed biopsychosocial approach increasingly powered by the neuroimmune science revolution. Graded Motor Imagery (GMI) is now a part of that revolution, not only as a series of novel treatment strategies, but also an increasing reminder that the representation of body in the brain should be considered in all patients. It also informs us that we (clinicians and patients) can and must lift our expectations of outcome.

Graded Motor Imagery is a complex series of treatments including graded left/right judgement exercises, imagined movements and use of mirrors targeting neuropathic pain problems. These problems include states such as complex regional pain syndrome (CRPS) where in the past there was little effective therapy to offer. But the GMI treatments (let's not call it a programme as they are not preset) are vulnerable to misuse. It can be hard work. The treatment requires careful tailoring to individual patients and cannot exist alone without education, interdisciplinary support and an effective therapeutic relationship.

This handbook is aimed at clinicians, those suffering with neuropathic pain, their friends and family and those who pay the bills. We have written this handbook because we know from basic sciences, clinical trials and repeated anecdotal reports that GMI is a worthwhile treatment. While it is a complex technique, we want you the user (clinician and patient) to do it as well as you can. Let's start by helping you build a platform of powerful knowledge on which to base the treatment.

1.1 KNOWLEDGE AND REASONING

Now Lorimer is a smart chap – you can see that by all his writings and research and musings and the fact that we have come far enough to write a GMI handbook is due to his research, the research work of those who came earlier[11,12,15] and the many who he has encouraged to research. I also know he gets a bit ratty with me for wanting to take research into the clinic as soon as possible. Researchers love to say 'this requires more research' after their papers, or 'this shouldn't be taken to the clinic just yet'. Such a cautious lot – And as if we can wait! There is other science however that we (patients and clinicians) can use and this is clinical reasoning science. Tim has had classical training and vast experience in clinical decision making related to the use of GMI and you can see this in his chapter. All contributors to this manual argue that in the absence of a great deal of research which guides clinical practice, we require a high level of clinical decision making skills to get the best out of GMI. In other words, for many chronic pain states we are a long way from having clear guidelines or a simple recipe to follow. For example, there are clear guidelines available for the management of diabetes or rheumatoid arthritis but this is not so for some of the persistent pain states that readers have to deal with. It is all made more difficult too, as the clinical presentations of people with persistent pains are so different. GMI interventions must be clinically reasoned from the best available clinical evidence from what the patient in front of you presents, what exists in the literature, continued test-retest of interventions and the clinician's intuition and experience. Some readers will have the skill to take research, be aware of its limitations and strengths, add it to patient specific information and construct an appropriate and measurable management strategy.

If you are a patient, you will also have to become a clinical reasoner and problem solver. You cannot be just a passive recipient of a treatment as if you were taking a pill. You and your health professional will need to work together on this journey. When you have a chronic pain state, you will only be with a health professional for about 0.1% of the time. You obviously have to be a self manager, a clinical thinker and a problem solver because the problem belongs to you and those close to you for the rest of the time.

This introductory chapter is about the process of gaining knowledge as part of effective treatment. This knowledge and the gaining of this knowledge is the real power behind the reasoning and GMI outcomes. While there are no trials available (yet) which support the notion that knowledge influences the outcomes of GMI, all contributors to this handbook believe that the amount, quality and use of knowledge is critical. While a positive relationship between knowledge and outcome may be common sense, it is also supported by studies which show that explaining biology such as we do in *Explain Pain*[1], can have a beneficial outcome on exercise[10]. GMI is a form of exercise of course, albeit exercise of synapses.

Let's look at this thing we call knowledge.

2. A SPECIAL KIND OF KNOWLEDGE FOR GMI USERS

The following section summarises what is in the handbook as well as the special kind of knowledge that we believe it would be advantageous for GMI users to have.

2.1 WHAT IS IN THE HANDBOOK?

This handbook is made up of five chapters. It is not necessary to read it from start to finish – you can begin anywhere, but each chapter is linked and offers something different and special. We propose that the information needed to assist users in getting the best possible outcome from the GMI process should include:

A. Information on how we learn. This is what this chapter is about. You might as well become a teacher as well as a neuroscientist!

B. Some science knowledge in the area of 'does it work' and 'how might it work'. You will find this in Lorimer's chapter. Although chapter 2 is written more for the rehabilitation professional, it is important that any GMI user is aware that GMI has scientific evidence for its use, both from clinical trials and basic sciences, and that this research continues. For the person in pain – the scientists are working for you. We suggest that patients read as much as they can and discuss some of the findings with their clinicians.

C. Some knowledge about how to perform GMI. Tim, in chapter 3 takes us through the clinical decision making process, including problem solving and progression of the therapy with 'real' patients. We want patients to become experts at their problem, not just the passive recipient of the treatment. This is so important as in many cases, the programme will take time, be intense and require problem solving along the way. Tim's chapter will help you to negotiate some of these corners.

D. Answers to common questions about the brain. I present this in chapter 4 and I have also included a section on metaphors and quotes that can help you along the way.

E. Some computer skills. The Recognise™ online and the Recognise App will be one of your greatest tools in the GMI programme. Tom has been working with the Recognise programme since its inception and he will take you through the nuts and bolts (or megs and bytes!) to help you get the most out of the online Recognise programme and the Smart Phone App in a stress-free way.

2.2 THE PARADIGMS THAT UNDERPIN OUR WORK

This special kind of knowledge for effective graded motor imagery also includes some updated health paradigms. You may as well know where our thinking comes from. Paradigms could be considered overarching frameworks of knowledge which guide research, reading, thinking and clinical practice. These paradigms include the neuroscience refreshed biopsychosocial approach[5] the neuromatrix paradigm[8,9] and the pain mechanisms paradigm. I doubt that there would be a GMI approach without these paradigms so let me tell you a little bit about them.

Biopsychosocial approaches are increasingly recognised as the way to go for persistent pain states as they not only take into account what has gone wrong in the body and the brain (the 'bio') they also incorporate the influence of psychological and social variables. In other words, the biopsychosocial approach not only looks at the disease or injury it also incorporates the illness as well – how the problem is 'lived'. It also takes into account that the problems we see in individual patients are to some degree a reflection of problems and issues in the community as a whole, for example, how pain is viewed by the community.

The neuromatrix paradigm allows access to the representation of our bodies and our lives in the brain. For now, think of phantom limb pain – the situation where a person experiences pain in fresh air, or the space where the limb once was. In this situation the limb is still represented in the brain, although distorted[4]. You will read about the neuromatrix and pain neurotags in the next chapter. We also take a lot of information from the pain sciences paradigm[6], where the study of pain has become a speciality. Much of this information is less than a decade old. It is a very special and new education which we are suggesting as a complement to the physical side of the GMI process. In fact we like to say that we now know more about how the brain works in the last ten years than the 1000 before it. Many health practitioners may not have this knowledge.

This new information includes understanding of brain pathways, brain plasticity, how pain and stress are 'made' by the brain, mirror neurones, and knowledge from the world of psychology and physiotherapy such as graded exposure to activity and frameworks for assessment. All this is included in the coming chapters. We are quite excited by this knowledge and we want those in trouble to get excited by it as well.

3. THE IDEA OF KNOWLEDGE AS CONTEXT

A context is the temporary environment of an action or planned action. All our behaviours are contextual. A list of suggested contexts such as time, place and emotion in which to perform the components of GMI is offered in Tim's chapter. Here in my chapter, the focus is on knowledge as context. We believe it is the most powerful (and often forgotten) context of all. For example, when you are stressed by the expectation of some impending important information, the action of breathing is different to your breathing when you have the information. In a neuroscience sense, it means that if you perform an action or think of an action as you will be doing in the GMI programme, the knowledge context of the action will influence which network of brain cells represent the action. That sounds complex! Said differently, you move more easily, function better and your brain has less need to make pain when you know what is going on with your body.

Knowledge is a very special context. It can be de-threatening, give meaning to your symptoms, provide explanations, help with compliance, allow problem solving, link to future goals, allow progression of treatment and it can be passed on to other people like a useful virus. GMI tools such as the Recognise online programme and the Mirror Box can be powerful, but the tools must somehow relate and fit with your beliefs and knowledge if the best outcomes are going to be achieved. Left/right discrimination and imagery are a bit abstract too, so a sound understanding is going to be helpful to make them real.

But first, some education science – in the following section, four key features of enriching your knowledge in the area of GMI are discussed.

4. SOME SCIENCE BEHIND GAINING KNOWLEDGE

4.1 KNOWLEDGE ENRICHMENT AND CONCEPTUAL CHALLENGES

Learning can be easy sometimes – as missing and novel bits of information are added to our existing knowledge frameworks, filling in the gaps and adding new bits. For example, information about the recently discovered mirror neurones in the brain, those neurones which fire when you watch someone move or think of moving (discussed in Lorimer's chapter) can fill in information gaps. This may explain why we feel tired after watching an action movie or how sometimes even thinking of moving can make you sensitive. It also provides a basis for imagery therapy where we try to exercise a part of the brain without 'turning on pain'.

But learning is often not easy – no one likes to be wrong and it can be uncomfortable when there are often challenges to our firmly held existing concepts, and other people offer competing theories. We are well aware that embarking on a GMI strategy is very likely to challenge existing concepts from both the patient and the therapist's perspectives and we want to help this. A big challenge for many patients is that they may have been told or it has been inferred that *'your pain is in your head'* (it ultimately is! It is your brain, not the rest of your body which decides whether pain is worth constructing). Another likely challenge is that we and hopefully other therapists will tell you that *'pain doesn't necessarily relate to tissue damage'* (it doesn't – some people have horrible injuries but report no pain). These challenges may be harder to deal with if the person has been told by an uninformed dinosaurial health professional that their 'pain is in their head', in a derogatory way. There is lots of unhelpful information and myths about pain out there in society, for example that *'you have to live with it'* (you don't) or *'you can't teach an old dog new tricks'* (you certainly can). We will deal with some of these unhelpful sayings later in the chapter and some readers may find *Explain Pain*[1] helpful when dealing with the key notions of 'your pain being in your head' and 'pain not necessarily relating to tissue damage'.

4.2 GRAINS OF UNHELPFUL AND INCORRECT INFORMATION

There is a lot of unhelpful information out there and some will require challenging. The unhelpful information that we all carry can be categorised into varying 'grain' sizes. Let's use sand as the metaphor[2] with the grain sizes ranging from single grains of sand to the sandcastle to solid chunks of sandstone (Figure 1.1).

The single grain

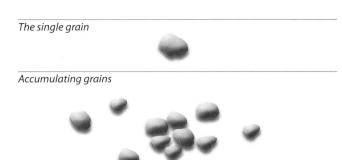

Accumulating grains

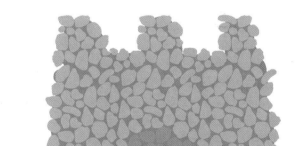

Formation of a sand castle

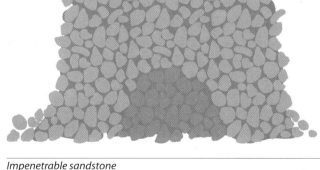

Impenetrable sandstone

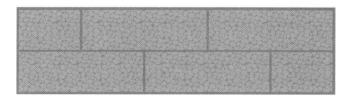

Figure 1.1 *The various 'grain' sizes of unhelpful information. Grains of unhelpful information can be at a singular grain level or grains can join together to form an unhelpful but changeable concept (sandcastle) or join together in a solid and difficult to change chunk of sandstone.*

At the single grain size are isolated pieces of unhelpful information that if you knew more about, or understood it better, life would be a bit easier. Examples of such information at the singular grain size include *'the brain won't change much in older people'*, (it surely will – our brains change all the time) or *'the health professional knows best'*, (not necessarily so as some are out of date) or that *'a scan is sure to find the cause'* (unlikely in persistent pain as there can be many causes, some of which can't be scanned, such as beliefs and feelings). We ask that all users continually seek what it is that they want to know or are not sure of. These days it is quite *likely* that science will have an answer or be working on an answer. With a bit of a challenge, sometimes argument, conceptual challenges at singular grain sizes can be easily dealt with as long as rational and understandable alternatives can be provided or sought out.

But often, people with persistent pain have unhelpful and wrong information at the conceptual level. Here, grains of unhelpful or wrong information have been collected and the grains are united under one conceptual banner, i.e. enough grains to form a sandcastle. For example, there may be a number of grains of information all united under the concept of *'I have pain therefore I am damaged'*. This will often be an important sandcastle to try to let a wave of learning wash over, as the amount of pain, especially chronic pain, rarely relates to damaged tissues. Some possible grains of information related to this concept have been suggested in Figure 1.2. Note that correct information can be held with grains of incorrect information and need liberating.

Figure 1.2 *Grains of unhelpful/incorrect information linking to form a sandcastle under the concept of 'I have pain therefore I must be damaged'.*

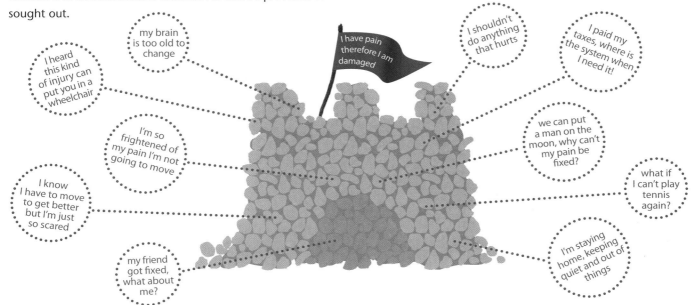

Other examples of potentially unhelpful concepts include *'this happened at work, work has to fix it'*, (an injury may well have happened at work and be related to worksite issues but ultimately work can't fix it, it is up to you and your health professionals). It is worth an analysis of the grains of beliefs and ideas which could make up the concept though. 'Grains' of anger directed at different people, blame apportioning, poor worksite practice, financial stress, links to other not quite unresolved injuries and ergonomic shortcomings can all contribute to the concept. A similar and linked concept here is *'I am going to keep looking until I can find someone who knows what is going on and who can fix it'*. This relentless search for a passive answer is known to be destructive, simply because there is usually no passive answer – in the vast majority of persistent pain states, an active reengagement with the 'self' is required. However it is quite understandable why this concept could persist (*'my friend was fixed, what about me; medicine is good enough for heart transplants, why can't it fix my back; I have paid my taxes, where is the system when I need it'*). Belief in the authority and power of medicine is often destroyed by the experience of persistent pain.

Another example of a common unhelpful/incorrect belief held at conceptual level is *'I shouldn't do anything that hurts'*. The answer here is that when pain is due more to changes in the nervous system rather than the processes that are associated with injured tissues, it is actually 'safe' to do activities which create a little bit of pain. The key of course is that the owner of the pain understands this. Tim discusses this in his chapter when he writes about graded

activity, I discuss it when I write about the twin peaks in chapter 4 and it is a key issue in *Explain Pain*[1].

It's hard to challenge strong, well constructed conceptual beliefs head on, for example to suddenly accept that *'Okay I have pain but I am not damaged'*. Or *'Okay it mightn't be all work'*. Each of the grains which make up these concepts should be identified where possible, addressed or challenged if possible. Thus it's not the concept which should be directly challenged but by picking away at the grains which make up the concept bit by bit, the concept may dissolve or weaken. As I have hinted, it is like a sand castle when the waves begin to lap the castle walls, nibbling away at them.

Finally, the grain level may be at complete paradigm level where multiple concepts link to form a distinct way of thinking which permeates many aspects of the person's life. It's more like sandstone than a sandcastle. Some may be culturally and religiously influenced. Examples may be a complete belief in passive treatment (such as surgery, drugs or massage) or a total belief in one particular health professional's direction. Even the classic Australian *'she'll be right mate, I don't want anyone to touch me'* can be hard to change. It is very difficult to change such thinking via education and it may be best to try to manage within that viewpoint if you are the clinician or to adapt GMI to fit your thinking if you are a patient.

4.3 DEEP KNOWLEDGE IS BETTER THAN SUPERFICIAL KNOWLEDGE

A central doctrine of educational theory is that learners can follow a deep or superficial learning pathway[7,14] (Figure 1.3). Use of the deep route is universally encouraged in education and we encourage it here.

The deep learning route involves systematic, thoughtful and deep information processing, so that the knowledge can ultimately being used as a coping strategy. The superficial pathway involves heuristics ('rules of thumb'), little thought or contemplation about information and sometimes even avoidance of issues. Conceptual change based on deep processing is regarded as superior to peripheral as it involves high levels of engagement, deeper understanding and continued learning. It places emphasis on an active role for the learner, to enable the use of knowledge as therapy.

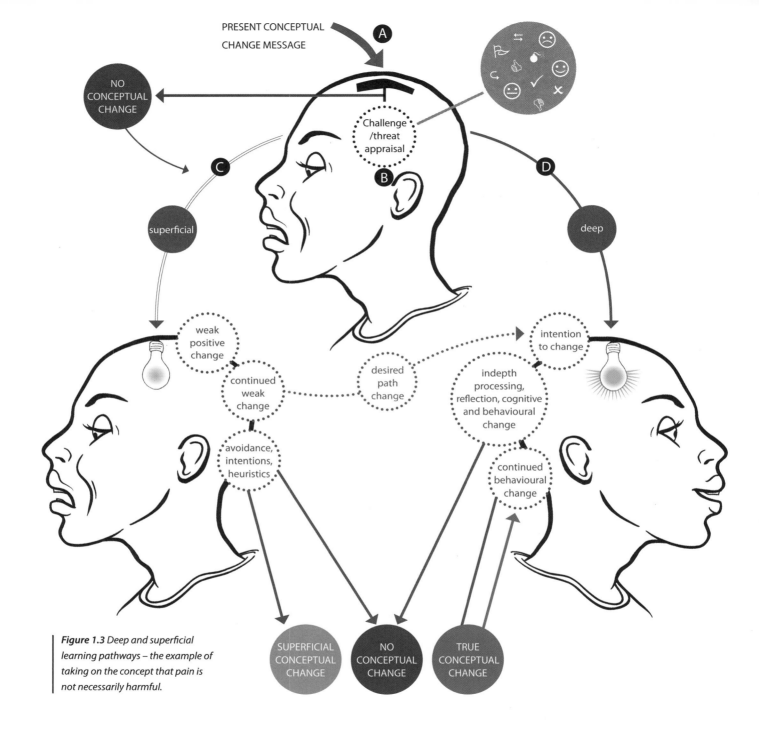

Figure 1.3 *Deep and superficial learning pathways – the example of taking on the concept that pain is not necessarily harmful.*

Let's go through the deep and superficial learning pathways by following the diagram.

A. Here the concept that pain does not always signal danger is presented. This is a critical piece of understanding to grasp for clinicians and patients with persistent pain. There will be many variables present which dictate what happens when this information is presented – variables related to you (for instance are you ready to listen?) the 'teacher' (for example, style of presentation), the message (or what format is used for delivery) and even the context (for instance is there a paying authority only allowing one visit?). Note in the diagram that there is a complete rejection route. We call this the 'bugger off route' (no conceptual change) where the patient will not even contemplate the information and may well walk out. Note the little arrow out of the box though – at another time and place he/she may listen.

B. At B, the person then decides to engage the information, but this could be in a number of ways – from varying degrees of interest, to a deep challenge. Here, even the information can hurt if it is a big enough challenge. We have sometimes heard patients say that reading *Explain Pain* hurts. This obviously wasn't the intention of the book but it does say something of the power of words. Note from B, there are two pathways of learning which follow, C, the peripheral learning route and D, the deep learning route. Let's follow C first.

C. Most of us take information superficially, at least in the first instance. It takes a lot of effort and resources to deeply process something such as *'pain doesn't necessarily mean damage'*. Taking this on superficially may simply mean not doing the graded activities suggested, avoiding the reading and the contemplation time. Sometimes it may even be putting off appointments and not giving the problem the priority it deserves and seeking out other health professionals who work in ways that match the beliefs about pain that you have always held. Those who follow a superficial pathway are unlikely to go onto much conceptual change with the information and it can be a waste of time for all.

D. We would obviously like you to be a deep learner and follow path D. Here is where the information is 'given a go' and the learner has decided, often with some help and support, that he or she is ready and confident to absorb the information about pain and to test the idea that pain does not necessarily signal damage. Unfortunately, such decisions to make a conceptual change are now very easily reversed. This could be due to competing information from the internet, a neighbour or an out of date health practitioner. However if you follow the path, with education and support, useful changes can occur. But the information has to be tested. This may mean doing a bit more activity, coaxing into pain, it may mean reflecting on the things which seem to increase the pain. Such reflection might include thoughts (*'am I worse when I'm upset?'*) or contexts (*'am I worse when in the presence of someone I don't like?'*). If successful and the information is taken on, deep learning will follow, other linked information will be more easily integrated and the information can be extrapolated to other aches and pains. Overall, deep learning produces longer lasting changes which are more resistant to counter argument than peripheral route processing[13]. However, note in Figure 1.3 that at the end of the deep learning pathway rejection can still happen. A common example is a personal campaign to stop smoking. It all seems to make sense and then something happens and you revert to smoking, or in the case of pain management, reject the management suggestion and seek something perhaps more instant such as surgery. All contributors to the book have mentioned 'patience and persistence, courage and commitment' and this is where it comes into your learning curve.

If you, the GMI user have deep knowledge about your problems and the process of GMI, it means you'll have skills to construct answers to questions such as *'why am I hurting so much today?'* and you'll be able to reason why you have good days and bad days. For example, knowledge of the biological influences of fearful thoughts and contexts (such as *why am I hurting more at work?*) may provide an answer. With deep knowledge, you'll have skills to progress treatment and you'll know when to back off treatment (see the patient examples in Tim's chapter). With deep knowledge, you'll be aware of new research (and be able to judge its quality) and you may be a very useful member of health related blog sites if you wish to be. Deep learning is the ability to use knowledge to self analyse and make change. When a person has a sensitive, easily fired up pain problem, every input such as a movement or a thought defaults to pain. With a brain that is empowered by knowledge, this may not be the case.

4.4 'OUT OF THE SHADOWS LEARNING'

We believe that this is an important concept for all users personally and for the overall development of the GMI process. Flagged by diSessa[3] it is a concept where a minor intuitive idea or a finding that has not been previously linked to the GMI process becomes important in the development of GMI, either for an individual or for the overall process. The knowledge about GMI is still 'in pieces' to some degree, so 'out of the shadows learning' and understanding is very likely to happen and we would like to know about it.

If you read NOI notes on 'By George', www.noigroup.com/ notes, the man who veered right while walking and was found to have a foot left/right discrimination deficit, you have a classic example of 'out of the shadows' learning. George would say that he 'couldn't find his feet in the morning'. We could make some sense of the right sided veering for George and we now research for left/right discrimination deficits in a range of central nervous system problems. In the past, patients have reported how stress could affect their left/right discrimination scores or how wrist stiffness post Colle's fracture immobilisation could be helped with mirror therapy. Some users have reported back on the design of the Recognise programme or shape of the mirror box and it has all been very helpful.

We do hear some weird stuff, in fact we love hearing about weird stuff. We want you to know that you are not going crazy. In his chapter, Tom tells readers the best way to report back and bring your findings 'out of the shadows' and to our attention. When we hear of patterns of responses, it directs our research interests.

5. A KNOWLEDGE CONTRACT

When you are seeking knowledge, a form of 'contract' can help. This contract is something you can make with yourself or with a health professional. The basic information that a person will probably want to know when he or she is in trouble, particularly in pain, can be put into four questions:

- What is wrong with me?
- How long will it take?
- What can I do for it?
- What can other health professionals do for it?

I guess you may also want to know how much it will all cost, but overall, if you are a patient reading this, make sure these questions are answered. If you are a health professional we suggest that you try your best to work together with your patient to provide the answers. This handbook will provide some of the answers – you may need to seek out other resources such as *Explain Pain* for information.

You may also ask yourself whether you are ready to take on the programme and how confident you are that you can give it your best. These are issues to be discussed with your health professional. If you can uncover and deal with any obstacles to progress before you get going, all the better. The more knowledge you have, the easier this will be.

REFERENCES

1. Butler DS, Moseley GL. *Explain Pain*. Adelaide: Noigroup Publications, 2003.

2. Chi MTH. Three types of conceptual change: Belief revision, mental model transformation and categorical shift. In Vosniadou S ed. International Handbook of Research on Conceptual Change. New York: Routledge, 2008.

3. diSessa AA. A bird's-eye view of the 'pieces' vs 'coherence' controversy. In Vosniadou S ed. International Handbook on Research on Conceptual Change. New York: Routledge, 2008.

4. Flor H, Devor M, Jensen T. Phantom limb pain: Causes and cures. In Dostrovsky JO, Carr DB, Kolzenburg M eds. Progress in Pain Research and Management. Seattle: IASP Press, 2003.

5. Gatchel RJ, Peng YB, Peters ML, et al. The biopsychosocial approach to chronic pain: Scientific advances and future directions. Psychological Bulletin 2007;133:581-624.

6. Gifford L, Butler D. The integration of pain sciences into clinical practice. The Journal of Hand Therapy 1997;10:86-95.

7. Gregoire M. Is it a challenge or a threat? A dual-process model of teacher's cognition and appraisal process during conceptual change. Educational Psychology Reviews 2005;15:117-55.

8. Melzack R. Pain and the neuromatrix in the brain. Journal of Dental Education 2001;65:1378-82.

9. Moseley GL. A pain neuromatrix approach to rehabilitation of chronic pain patients. Man Ther 2003;8:130-40.

10. Moseley GL, Hodges PW, Nicholas MK. A randomized controlled trial of intensive neurophysiology education in chronic low back pain. Clinical Journal of Pain 2004;20:324-30.

11. Nico D, Daprati E, Rigal F, et al. Left and right hand recognition in upper limb amputees. Brain 2004;127:120-32.

12. Parsons LM. Integrating cognitive psychology, neurology and neuroimaging Acta Psychologica 2001;107:155-81.

13. Petty RE, Cacioppo JT, Sedikides C, et al. Affect and persuasion: a contemporary perspective. The American Behavioural Scientist 1988;31:355-71.

14. Piaget J. The equilibration of cognitive structures. Chicago: University of Chicago Press, 1985.

15. Schwoebel J, Coslett HB, Bradt J, et al. Pain and the body schema: effects of pain severity on mental representations of movement. Neurology 2002;59:775-7.

NOTES

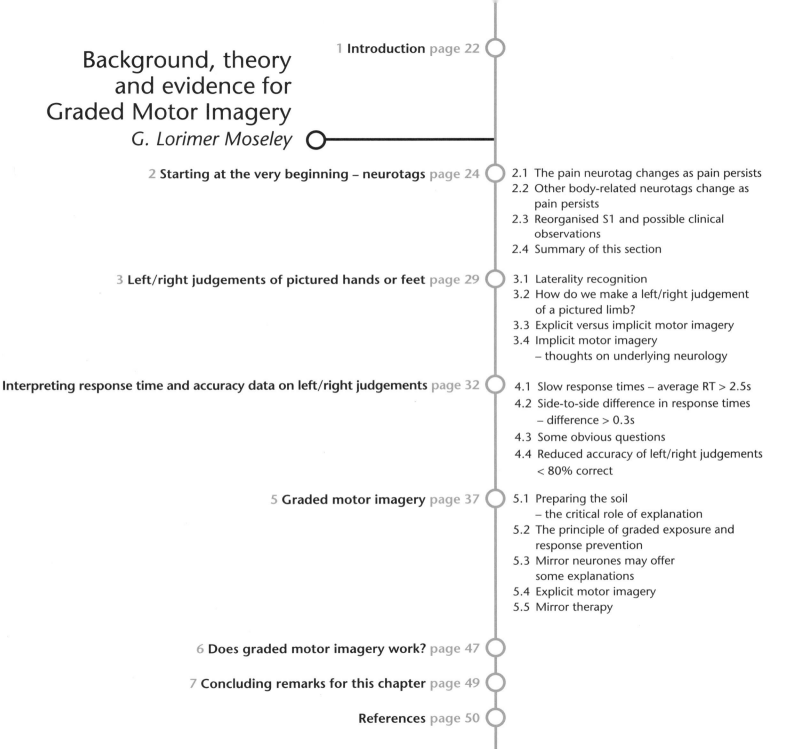

Background, theory
and evidence for
Graded Motor Imagery
G. Lorimer Moseley

1. INTRODUCTION

After physiotherapy school, I spent a while knocking about in the Australian bush, delaying the start of what I then thought would be a fairly unremarkable career going through the motions of fixing people in pain. How ridiculously naïve I was! When the gap between my income, as a second rate muso and part-time tutor and the cost of living, primarily on lentil soup and vegemite sandwiches, became too large, I took up a physiotherapy job at the New South Wales Academy of Sport in my home town of Sydney. I soon realised that not only was it difficult to help someone in chronic pain, I did not even understand why they were in pain in the first place! There might be no evidence that the body tissues themselves were still damaged. Their pain might jump around with no apparent relationship to anything they did. Their pain might be severe, debilitating and ruthless, but their injury nothing more than a mild sprain. This gradual realisation, that pain was about more than the state of the tissues, presented me with a difficult dilemma – how on earth should we go about treatment?

I wrestled with that dilemma clinically for a few years, until I came across a dog-eared, scuffed up and scrawled-over copy of *Phantoms in the brain*[40] by the effusive neurologist Vilayanur Ramachandran. Aside from being a very enjoyable read, it was a well-timed read too – I began reading it midway up the glorious New South Wales north coast on a road trip that I had planned to coincide with the only conference I could possibly justify as relevant to my work. I turned up for my single session – not wanting to submit

the receipts to the tax office without ever having attended. I sat myself down in the front row. I remember being struck at how many women were wearing sensible shoes and how many men wore polo shirts. I was barefoot as I recall.

The first speaker was a balding fellow with bright green glasses and red jeans. 'Courageous' I thought. He was a great speaker, yet he was almost being booed off stage for making the outrageous suggestion, over and over again, that a patient's brain might be a useful ally in the quest for pain relief. Then he called us all possums and I giggled out loud. In a matter of a couple of days, I had met these two clinicians who seemed to be singing from a different songsheet to the rest of us. They were making very profound suggestions. Suggestions that were loaded with substantial challenges, confronting realities and exciting opportunities. My rapidly waning relationship with rehabilitation was reignited such that now, nigh on twenty years later, I am still gobsmacked at the fearful and wonderful complexity of the human and the seemingly endless opportunities to recruit the very thing that Vilayanur Ramachandran and David Butler so outrageously suggested to be worthy of consideration – the brain.

Among other anecdotes and clinical accounts, Ramachandran's book described the response of a patient with phantom limb pain when he put his hand behind a mirror and moved 'both' hands. He watched the reflection of his intact hand, which moved perfectly well and was exactly where he felt his phantom limb to be. The phantom 'came alive'[40]. The patient was, it seemed, miraculously cured of his chronic phantom limb pain. I recall this to be as complete and instant a cure as one could ever want to induce. I have only seen it happen like that once. I witnessed an amputee being kidnapped by his Doctor. The doctor injected him with something to put him to sleep and then strapped him to a seat. I saw this happen. When the patient returned to consciousness, he was sitting in front of a mirror. The Doctor forced him to put his intact arm in front of the mirror and his phantom arm behind the mirror and look into the mirror. There, in full view, was his phantom arm – alive! Shibang! Cured. That was the last episode I ever watched of the television series *House*.

Ramachandran's account was less dramatic than Dr House's experience, but it was still pretty remarkable and it motivated me to get a mirror and try it. I tried it on everyone with leg or arm pain. The results were, out of memory, sometimes excellent, sometimes horrible. One clinical condition that seemed well suited to the mirror and which completely fascinated me, was complex regional pain syndrome (CRPS). To be honest, as a physiotherapist, I had been able to offer people with CRPS absolutely nothing that seemed helpful. With mirror in hand, I stumbled along with a few great outcomes and many shocking ones – nothing all that different from what I would expect from any kind of treatment.

This seemingly hopeless situation was of immediate interest to me – I like the idea of biting off more than I can chew and then chewing like hell. I became more and more enamored with the role of the brain in chronic pain. I started a PhD with Mr-Transversus-Abdominis Paul Hodges. I started to read about motor imagery. I began playing with motor imagery in treatments and while some of the trickier patients seemed to respond well, some were aggravated by imagined movements! How do you get less threatening than imagined movements? I then stumbled across a research article by a group in Philadelphia, USA. The paper reported delayed reaction time in a left/right hand judgement task in people with hand pain[42]. Therein lies the start of my involvement in the journey towards graded motor imagery. It is not my brain-child but I do not know anyone who has found it quite as fascinating nor perplexing as I have.

GMI
hand
book

2. STARTING AT THE VERY BEGINNING – NEUROTAGS

I do not know how the brain works. I am pretty sure that no one does. What I do know is that the people who seem to know the most about how the brain works seem to love this idea – that the brain represents things. We often call these representations, cortical representations, 'maps' or 'neurotags'[2]. I like the last one – neurotag. A neurotag is a network of interconnected neurones, we will call brain cells, that are distributed throughout the brain. When a neurotag is activated it produces an output. The output defines

the neurotag. For example, the neurotag for neck pain refers to the network of brain cells that, when activated, produces neck pain. The neurotag for the smell of bread is that network of brain cells that, when activated, produces the smell of bread. Crucial here is that the smell-of-bread neurotag does not produce the odour itself, nor does it detect it. Rather, it produces the experience of smelling the bread (Figure 2.1A,B).

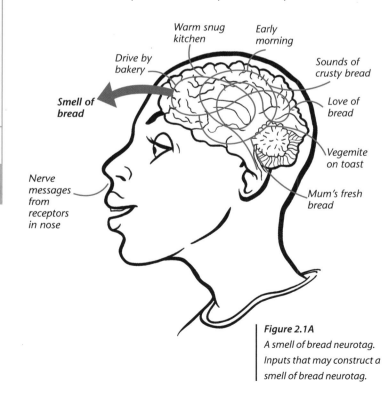

Warm snug kitchen

Early morning

Drive by bakery

Sounds of crusty bread

Smell of bread

Love of bread

Vegemite on toast

Nerve messages from receptors in nose

Mum's fresh bread

Figure 2.1A
A smell of bread neurotag.
Inputs that may construct a
smell of bread neurotag.

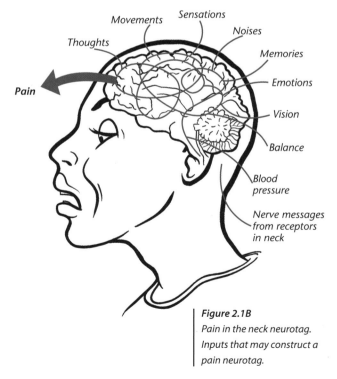

Movements

Sensations

Noises

Thoughts

Memories

Emotions

Pain

Vision

Balance

Blood pressure

Nerve messages from receptors in neck

Figure 2.1B
Pain in the neck neurotag.
Inputs that may construct a
pain neurotag.

The timing of activation of the brain cells that make a neurotag is almost certainly very important but scientists do not have a method by which to measure the timing of individual brain cells. Although brain imagers are starting to be excited about the connectedness of our brains[43], this is a bit different and the best we can do at the moment is to take an educated guess. This is the guess: that the brain cells have to fire in a certain pattern. For now, we can say that they have to fire together – as one. We know a bit more about where the brain cells that make up a neurotag might be, although brain cells are so small that we can not be any more precise than locating them to the nearest several thousand brain cells. These limitations are important physiologically, but I do not think that they are important conceptually.

What is important conceptually is that to activate any particular neurotag, two criteria have to be met:

1. The member brain cells have to fire. That is, the neurones that make up the neurotag have to fire.

2. Nearby brain cells have to NOT fire. If non-member brain cells fire, the neurotag is changed, is imprecise, is wrong if you like.

Neurotags can be considered as having an activation threshold, much like individual brain cells (in fact all neurones in the body) have. For individual brain cells, the activation threshold is the level of excitement at which the brain cell 'fires'. For neurotags, the activation threshold is the level of excitement at which the neurotag is activated and produces its output. Neurotags, like individual brain cells, can have changing levels of excitement below their

activation threshold. This is an important concept because each of the member brain cells is itself open to modulation by other brain cells with which it communicates. This is a very useful way of understanding how a potentially infinite number of factors can modulate a given pain neurotag.

2.1   THE PAIN NEUROTAG CHANGES AS PAIN PERSISTS

There is now a huge number of research articles that describe the substantial changes in function and structure that occur in the central nervous system when pain persists. The vast majority of these articles focus their attention on the spinal cord – in particular the neurones that transmit a danger message from the spinal cord to the brain (if you want to learn more about these changes, see[45] for a review). Over the last decade or two, scientists have expanded their focus to unravel a range of changes in the brain as well as the spinal cord. It is beyond me and not within the scope of this book to review all of those changes here - the interested reader is referred to more focused reviews[8,13,25,44]. Let's focus instead on the nature of the changes that occur in the pain neurotag.

When pain persists, the pain neurotag becomes *sensitised* and *disinhibited*. *Sensitisation* of the pain neurotag refers to an increase in the excitability of the member brain cells such that they are more easily activated. The principle of this increase in excitability is the same as that of individual neurones that become potentiated, or 'wound-up'. Sensitisation of the pain neurotag is like the whole network of brain cells being 'wound-up'. Sensitisation of

C 2
2 5
www.noigroup.com
Background, theory and evidence of Graded Motor Imagery
GMI hand book

the pain neurotag offers the most sensible explanation as to why, as pain persists, pain is evoked more easily and by a wider array of internal and external stimuli than it is initially. Remember a couple of pages back, I recalled being exasperated that even imagined movements made some patients worse. As a physiotherapist I was left pondering how we can get under the radar of a pain neurotag that is so sensitive that it is even activated by the intent to move. This is where left/right judgements come in, but more of that in a moment.

Remember that for a neurotag to be activated, it requires sufficient activation of the member brain cells and sufficient inhibition of the non-member brain cells? Well, *disinhibition* refers to a decrease in this inhibition of non-member brain cells. This sounds complex but it just means that they're not dampened down. Perhaps an easier way to think about it is to say that the neurotags lose precision. This effect probably only involves neurotags that are relevant to the pain neurotag. Disinhibition might manifest as spreading pain, pain that moves, pain that is less precisely defined anatomically or qualitatively. The pattern of spread will not adhere to the distribution of a peripheral nerve, or to that of a nerve root. Instead, pain will spread to a whole limb, a body region or to a whole side of the body. Disinhibition of movement neurotags will manifest as imprecise movements or perhaps in the extreme, dystonia.

Let's make one more return to that troublesome observation of pain on imagined movements. Both disinhibition and sensitisation might contribute to pain on imagined movements. Let's say one imagines writing the letter 'G'.

When one writes 'g' in a disinhibited state, the 'g' comes out messier than it normally would. This will also be the case when one simply imagines writing 'g' while in a disinhibited state. The actual and imagined movements are both imprecise[1]. Now, if the hand pain neurotag is highly sensitised, the disinhibition might be sufficient to 'set off' the hand pain neurotag. So, pain on imagined writing might be a result of disinhibition AND sensitisation. Either way, left/right judgements are a sensible thing to do to turn around the pain neurotag – but hang on, we are getting there.

2.2 OTHER BODY RELATED NEUROTAGS CHANGE AS PAIN PERSISTS

Disinhibition is the most likely explanation for the range of body-related neurotags that can become disrupted as pain persists. The most investigated of these involves an area of the brain called the primary sensory cortex, or S1. S1 sits in the outermost layer of your brain, which makes it particularly easy to investigate. By placing recording electrodes on the outside of the skull, it is possible to detect changes in activity in S1.

1. Doing this experiment will help explain the fact that imagined writing will be messier in a disinhibited state: stand 20m from a wide open door and time how long it takes to imagine walking from where you are, through the door and back again. Now close the door a bit so it is a narrow opening, although you can still squeeze through. Time yourself doing it again. Did you notice that the second time is slower? This is because your imagining the task depends on the characteristics of the movements required. So too, if your writing is messy because you have had hand pain for 5 years, your imagined writing becomes messier too.

Scientists also investigate S1 using functional magnetic brain imaging (fMRI), which can detect changes in blood oxygen levels throughout the brain, not just in the outermost layer. Either method can be used to investigate which S1 brain cells are involved in the 'feeling-something-on-my-skin' neurotag.

The organisation of S1 is fairly consistent between people, which means that we can be reasonably confident that if we stimulate the pinky on our right hand, we will see a nice activation in a particular location in the left S1. If we stimulate the fourth finger on our right hand, we will see a nice activation just next door to the activation caused by stimulating the pinky. If we stimulate the index finger it will be slightly further away again. The pattern of activation that emerges when we keep stimulating different spots on the skin is called the sensory homunculus. Much has been written about the sensory homunculus (Figure 2.2) – almost without exception it involves men so we actually know very little about the female sensory homunculus – we presume it is the same except for the obvious differences! I won't review all that writing here, but I will focus on the changes in the sensory homunculus that have been observed in people with persistent pain.

Most data are from patients with phantom limb pain or CRPS. In those conditions, the area of S1 that corresponds to the hand decreases. That is, in CRPS the distance between the activation caused by stimulating the pinky and the activation caused by stimulating the thumb is decreased[14]. Of course it is impossible to stimulate a phantom finger, so scientists stimulate the lip, which is

the 'next in line' in S1 homonculus. In finger amputees with phantom limb pain, stimulating the lip activates S1 brain cells that are in what is normally the hand area of the homonculus. In amputees without phantom limb pain, it does not[7]. Collectively, these changes in how the brain cells in the S1 homonculus respond to sensory stimuli are termed 'cortical reorganisation'. Disinhibition causes cortical reorganisation and although there are also probably other processes involved, disinhibition is the process that is most relevant to us here.

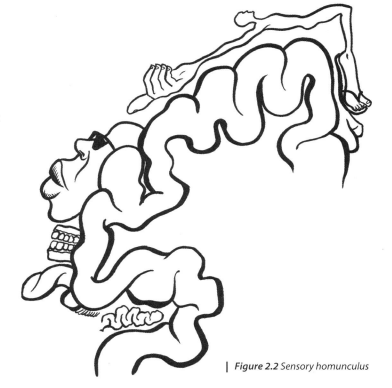

| *Figure 2.2* Sensory homunculus

There are also data from patients with back pain. With this group, a different pattern has emerged – the area of S1 that is activated when the skin of the back is stimulated *increases* instead of decreases. It also moves[6]. We do not really know why the opposite sort of thing happens in back pain. But conveniently, the functional effect is in some ways similar – S1 becomes 'smudged', for example some S1 brain cells become activated when the left side of your back is touched AND when the right side of your back is touched. This means that touching the left side of your back might activate the 'touched-on-the-left-side-of-your-back' neurotag, or the 'touched-on-the-right-side-of-your-back' neurotag, or both. Can you see how this might make it difficult to know where a sensory input is coming from?

2.3   REORGANISED S1 AND POSSIBLE CLINICAL OBSERVATIONS

There are two clinical observations that are most likely when S1 becomes reorganised. First, our sensation in the painful area becomes less precise. This is different to being numb or having a loss of sensory transmission. Experiments show that sensory transmission does not explain the problem but that these brain changes do. Clinicians can test this by measuring how far apart the stimuli have to be for the patient to detect two separate stimuli instead of one. This distance is called the two point discrimination threshold. The second clinical observation is that the perceived size and shape of the body part changes. These perceptual distortions are well recognised in amputees – the feeling

of a clenched fist and the feeling of an arm extended and abducted are particularly common in traumatic upper limb amputees[15,16]. People with CRPS tend to overestimate the size of their affected limb[18,19] and people with low back pain find it difficult to distinguish the outline of their trunk, or to differentially move their pelvis and back[22].

2.4 SUMMARY OF THIS SECTION:

- Neurotags are networks of brain cells that, when activated produce an output.

- For a neurotag to be activated, there needs to be sufficient activation of the member brain cells and inhibition of the adjacent non-member brain cells.

- The brain changes when pain persists – the pain neurotag becomes more sensitive and body-related neurotags lose their normal inhibition.

- Sensitisation results in: more pain and more easily evoked pain.

- Disinhibition results in: a loss of precision which can disrupt movement commands, sensory function, perception of the body part and anything else related to that body part.

3. LEFT/RIGHT JUDGEMENTS OF PICTURED HANDS OR FEET

3.1 LATERALITY RECOGNITION

Neurologically speaking, judging a pictured limb as belonging to one side of the body or the other is not a trivial task. There is a very large amount of research on this, most of it done by a fellow called Professor Laurie Parsons - you can sidestep most of the literature by reading his excellent review of it[39]. Early on these judgements were called 'laterality recognition'[28] but using this term caused a real problem with brainiacs who always use the term 'laterality' to describe where in the brain a functional centre resides. Using 'laterality' also caused headaches for the cognitive psychologists who talk about abilities as being lateralised (for example, artistic ability is thought to be *lateralised* to the right hemisphere). I have responded to their suggestions and tried to avoid the term 'laterality' when talking about left/right judgements. To do so is not wrong it is just problematic if we are talking with medics and cognitive psychologists.

Conventional uses of the term 'laterality' – top level tennis players who do not use a double handed backhand, for example the sublime Roger Federer, almost certainly has a right forearm that is very much larger than his left. He can be said to be lateralised in this regard. Females are, as a general rule, more lateralised in function than men – that is, they are more 'handed', but they are less lateralised neurologically and may be completely unlateralised morphologically. Starting to sound confusing? This is why I think we should stick with 'left/right judgements', or 'implicit motor imagery', instead of 'laterality' because then we avoid the risk of being misunderstood. However, 'laterality recognition' is now pretty well 'in' as a term, so you have my official permission to use it.

GMI hand book

3.2 HOW DO WE MAKE A LEFT/RIGHT JUDGEMENT OF A PICTURED LIMB?

Professor Parsons' work presents a very compelling argument that left/right judgements involve three distinct processes. The first is an immediate, spontaneous and unconscious judgement. The second is a mental movement by which we manoeuvre the body part in our mind by using some of the same brain neurotags that we would use to actually move the body part. If that mental movement confirms the initial judgement then we respond accordingly. If that mental movement does not confirm the initial judgement, then we start again. The middle step of this process seems to offer a sensible answer to that exasperated question I posed earlier – '*How can anything be less threatening than imagined movements?*' Left/right judgements clearly offer a possibility which we will explore now.

3.3 EXPLICIT VERSUS IMPLICIT MOTOR IMAGERY

When we first make left/right judgements, we are often aware that we are imagining the movement that allows us to confirm our initial judgement. If we are aware of this, then we are doing *explicit motor imagery*, or imagined movements. The more we practise, the less we realise that we are moving our own hand in our brain – brain imaging studies suggest it takes about 40 judgements, although it varies a lot between people[25]. Even though we no longer explicitly imagine the movement, we are still mentally moving our own limb – we just do not know that we are. Once we are at this stage, we are doing *implicit motor imagery*.

Explicit motor imagery can exacerbate pain and swelling in people with CRPS[23,29,37], in people with non-CRPS hand pain[37] and in people with pain related to spinal cord injury[9]. Anecdotally, those with chronic back or neck pain sometimes report that imagined back or neck movements can aggravate their pain, but to my knowledge this phenomenon has not been systematically investigated in these groups. Nonetheless there is no reason to predict that spinal pain would behave differently to non-spinal pain in this regard. That explicit motor imagery can exacerbate pain suggests that we should inform the patient of this possibility, but in a manner that dethreatens the task.

> *Experience suggests:* Explain to patients that left/right judgements can aggravate symptoms initially, that this is transient and almost certainly related to sensitive brain networks associated with movement. Once the brain learns how to do this task without imagining the movement, the pain is unlikely to be aggravated.

Anecdotally, my own experience suggests that fully explaining the process that is involved in left/right judgements can impede its effect. This was at first perplexing and counter to my own commitment as part of rehabilitation to give patients the resources to master their situation – I try to give them as much understanding as they can take. My suspicion was that by telling patients that their brain is mentally moving their body even when they do not *feel* it, we were introducing a threat, possibly associated with movement or with a reduced sense of control. According to the whole neurotag sensitisation issue discussed earlier, it is very possible that this information actually increased the excitement of the pain neurotag in those people for whom any type of movement was highly threatening (for more on this sort of thing, see *Explain Pain*[2]).

> *Experience suggests: Do not emphasise the role of motor processes in left/right judgements. Perhaps instead emphasise the role of refining body related neurotags in a non-threatening manner.*

3.4   IMPLICIT MOTOR IMAGERY – THOUGHTS ON UNDERLYING NEUROLOGY

One aspect of implicit motor imagery that warrants special mention concerns its underlying neurology. Movement involves many brain areas. The area of the brain that seems most involved in intentional movement is called the Primary Motor Cortex – it sits just across a crevice (called a sulcus) from S1 (the Primary Sensory Cortex, remember?) and is called, conveniently, M1. Explicit motor imagery (or 'imagined movements') involves activation of brain cells in M1 in a manner similar to that involved in actually doing the movement[4,5]. However, implicit motor imagery (or left/right judgements) does not[35]. Implicit motor imagery does activate an area known as the Premotor Cortex, which is important in the planning of movements and is known to send messages to specific M1 cells that will be involved with the movement (See table 2.1). That is, premotor brain cells can cause changes in the excitement of M1 cells without activating them. This is a terrific situation for us for two reasons. First, it gives a mechanism by which we can expose the brain

cells of the pain neurotag to changes in excitement level without triggering the whole response (pain). Second, it lets us increase inhibition of non-member cells in body-related neurotags. So, we are potentially addressing both of the problems that occur when pain persists – we are decreasing sensitisation and normalising inhibition.

Implicit motor imagery (left/right judgements)	Explicit motor imagery (imagined movements)
You don't know you are mentally moving	You know you are mentally moving
Premotor cells modify primary motor cells without activating them	Primary motor cells are activated
Less likely to activate the pain neurotag	More likely to activate the pain neurotag

Table 2.1 Differences between explicit and implicit motor imagery

Let's return now to the process of making left/right judgements. The Recognise programme provides an excellent way to assess how well people make left/right judgements of body parts. Tom discusses the practical use of Recognise in chapter 5. For the moment however, it is important to know that you can take two pieces of information from a left/right judgement task – how fast you are (response time for making correct judgements) and how accurate you are. You are given separate response time and accuracy results for pictures of the left and right hands (or feet or back rotation or whatever Recognise body part you are working on). The key question then, from my perspective, is what do these results actually mean?

4. INTERPRETING RESPONSE TIME AND ACCURACY DATA ON LEFT/RIGHT JUDGEMENTS

The research on left/right judgements is still underway but a large number of studies have already been done. The following interpretations are sensible based on what we now know about the task. There are likely to be exceptions and individual performances are open to many variables, so it is best to consider these interpretations as general rules. There are several ways in which left/right judgements can be disrupted – slow response times, side to side differences and reduced accuracy of left/right judgements (less than 80%).

4.1 SLOW RESPONSE TIMES – AVERAGE RT > 2.5s

Generally slow response times probably reflect impairment of central nervous system processing. Some people are just slow on complex response time tasks. Slow response times on left/right judgements could involve any of the underlying processes: processing of the visual image to make an initial judgement, the mental movement of the body parts or the pressing of the button to respond. To untangle these processes one could compare performance on different body parts, or on simple or more complex response time tasks.

4.2 SIDE-TO-SIDE DIFFERENCE IN RESPONSE TIMES – DIFFERENCE > 0.3s

In this situation, it would seem most likely that an error is occurring in the initial judgement or in the final response. That is, let us say that a left hand is shown but the initial judgement made by the participant is 'right'. The second process, which involves the brain using a neurotag of the body part and preparing to move it to the position shown in the picture in order to confirm that judgement, actually shows the judgement to be wrong. According to what is understood about the task, the mental movement is undertaken a second time, but this time a neurotag of the opposite limb is involved at the same time. Second time around, the initial judgement is confirmed and the final response is triggered. The result? An accurate but delayed response.

4.3 SOME OBVIOUS QUESTIONS

4.3.1 What would cause a delay in the initial response?
Relevant to this question is a range of experiments that show information processing biases in people with chronic pain. There are several types of biases that have been described, but one in particular is most relevant here. When a sensory stimulus, in this case a picture of a body part, is first evaluated and there is some ambiguity about its possible interpretation, the brain may exert an evaluative bias. The bias will almost certainly be based on meaning. For example, let us imagine that you have eaten at many Italian restaurants and you quite enjoy bantering with a young swarthy waiter smelling of garlic. Let us then

imagine that you are mugged by a swarthy man who smells of garlic. Next time you are approached by a swarthy man who smells of garlic, you are being presented with an ambiguous stimulus – is this a waiter with whom you can engage in friendly banter or is this a mugger from whom you should escape? It is possible that your brain will exert an evaluative bias such that you conclude, more often than not, that the stimulus represents a mugger. As a general rule potentially dangerous stimuli out-trump harmless stimuli, even if they are as pleasurable in your eyes as a young Italian waiter might be.

Let's return to the issue at hand, so to speak. Let's say you have just injured your left hand and it is painful. You are shown a picture of a hand. This picture is 'the stimulus'. You are required to respond to that stimulus by judging it to be a left or a right hand. The stimulus is a bit ambiguous – perhaps it is in a peculiar posture or it is a right hand emerging from the left side of the screen. You will tend to conclude that the stimulus is in fact a left hand because that is the hand in which your brain is slightly more interested[36]. The same evaluative bias occurs if you have not just injured your hand and it is not in fact painful BUT you expect it to become painful at any moment[11]. In these scenarios, you will have a longer RT to make a left/right judgement when the picture coincides with your UNaffected hand because there will be an increased likelihood that your initial judgement is wrong – you correct it in the process of mental movements (implicit motor imagery), but it takes longer for you to make the final response.

GMI
hand
book

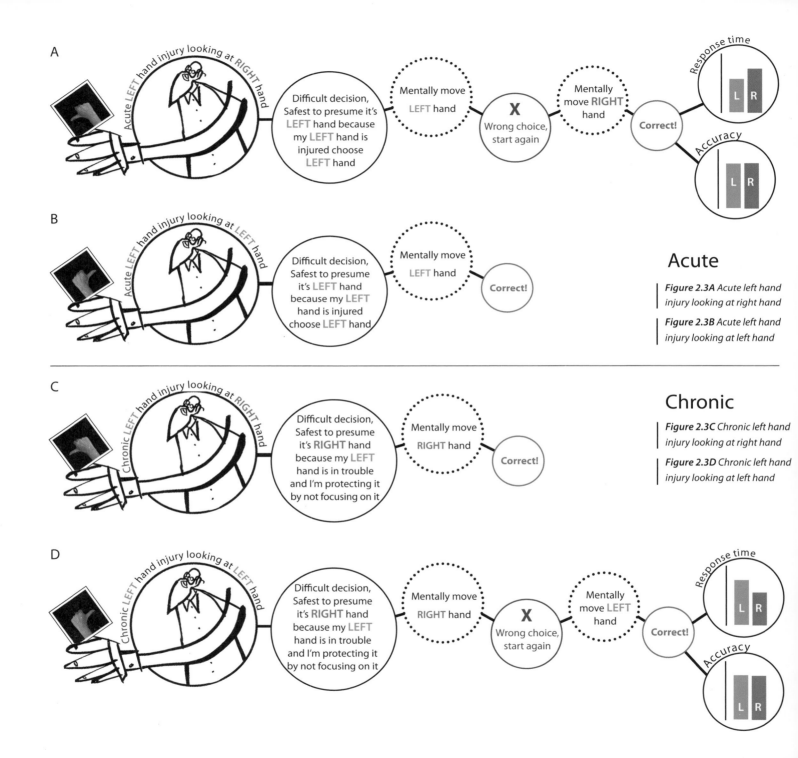

Acute

Figure 2.3A Acute left hand injury looking at right hand

Figure 2.3B Acute left hand injury looking at left hand

Chronic

Figure 2.3C Chronic left hand injury looking at right hand

Figure 2.3D Chronic left hand injury looking at left hand

4.3.2 How do you know it is a delay of one hand and not a speeding up of the other?

Based on what we know about how we make left/right judgements, it is not immediately obvious how they can be sped up other than by practice, or by some manipulation that enhances brain processing speed. For practice to have a side-specific effect, one would need to practice in front of images of one hand only. So as far as I know, it is safe to presume that a discrepancy in RT reflects a delay in decision making for images for one hand, not a speeding up of images for the other.

4.3.3 Why do patients usually have a delay on the painful hand?

I mentioned earlier a paper that alerted me to the left/right judgement task and delayed RT in people with arm pain[42]. That paper mentioned, almost in passing, that the patients had been diagnosed with CRPS. Since then, that finding has been replicated and extended[20,21,28], which means that it wasn't a quirky or erroneous finding. The most likely answer to this question has evolved as more studies have been conducted. I think the delay reflects an evaluative bias away from the painful hand, (that is, the RT score of the non-painful hand was lower than that of the painful hand, see Figure 2.3C) rather than an evaluative bias towards the painful hand (which is what we see in acute hand pain, see Figure 2.3A).

My reasons for this are: There is a building literature that CRPS in particular and chronic pain states in general, are associated with changes in spatial and somatotopic representation of body-related stimuli – a situation we have described elsewhere[30]. In short, this means that some of the neurotags that represent the anatomy of the body (somatotopic representations) and the space around the body (spatial representations) become disrupted, probably because of disinhibition. If you are remotely interested in this stuff and can take on a bit of a heavy article on it, we have written a paper that proposes the idea of a brain-held body-space matrix, that integrates not just maps of the body, but also regulation and protection of the body[30]. As with all such ideas, this one is a descendent of more established theories, for example the neuromatrix theory by Ron Melzack[13], and a theory that incongruence between motor and sensory output causes pathological pain[10] (although that theory has not been clearly supported by subsequent investigations – the jury is still out I guess; see[25] and[33,34]). Our idea of a cortical body matrix extends well beyond sensory-motor integration to cover the suite of bodily systems that can be disrupted in a range of neurological and psychiatric conditions, including chronic pathological pain.

The *cortical body matrix* is an integrated 'network of networks' that is responsible for surveillance, regulation, proprioception and perception of the body and its surrounding space. The part of all this that is relevant to GMI is that, in chronic pain, there seems to be a bias in tactile processing away from the painful body part, (better results for the non-painful body part) just like there is a bias away from the painful body part in left/right judgements which do not involve tactile input. Here is the twist though: remarkably, this bias is not specific to the body part in question but the space that the body part normally occupies – it can be reversed in unilateral arm pain by crossing both hands over the body midline[32]. For unilateral back pain, the bias is observed for stimuli applied to the back, but also for stimuli applied to the hands when the hands are held near the back. So, the stimulus arrives at the brain via sensory pathways unrelated to the back but the brain still prioritises away from the painful 'space'[38].

4.3.4 Why would the brain prioritise AWAY from the affected body part?

At this stage, we can only theorise about this. There are again two most likely explanations. The first is that the delayed RT reflects some kind of implicit attempt to reduce the provocation of pain. I am not completely settled on this idea because, after all, the brain is producing the pain and can choose not to produce pain even at times of massive spinal nociceptive barrage. The second is that it is just a mistake that occurs because the brain's maps of space are disrupted. At the moment this explanation feels better to me, but further experiments are required to untangle this one. Regardless of why it happens, it does seem to happen. An example of what might happen with someone with CRPS of one hand is shown in Figure 2.3D.

4.3.5 How does practising left/right judgements improve such an evaluative bias?

There is good evidence that practising left/right judgements reduces the delay in RT[20,21,24]. I have seen this happen within a session and I have seen it take a few weeks. According to our current understanding of what the delayed RT reflects, it seems reasonable to suggest that reduction of the delay reflects correction of the evaluative bias that causes it, or

of the disruption of spatial representation that I mentioned above. Again, we need to do more experiments to find out the neurological mechanisms that underpin it. It is tempting to conclude that, because reduction of the delay coincides with reduction of pain, then whatever is causing the delay is also causing the pain. This may be true, but it may be false. We simply do not know yet.

4.4 REDUCED ACCURACY OF LEFT/RIGHT JUDGEMENTS < 80% CORRECT

In this situation, it seems most likely that the ability of the brain to mentally move the limb in order to mimic the posture of the limb shown in the picture is impaired. The most likely explanation for this impairment is decreased precision of the neurotags of the limb, or a problem integrating the neurotag with the preparation for movement. At the moment I think the most likely explanation is the first one – there is a growing body of evidence that neurotags of the body are disrupted in chronic pain – see above and see reviews in the literature[8,13,25,44].

5. GRADED MOTOR IMAGERY

5.1 PREPARING THE SOIL – THE CRITICAL ROLE OF EXPLANATION

It would come as no surprise to anyone familiar with *Explain Pain*[2] that I take very seriously the role we have as educators. We are 'the voice of a thousand scientists'. I am firmly convinced that people in pain do better if they are given the resources to master their situation. In order to do this, I think they should understand as much as they can and have realistic expectations about the extent and time course of rehabilitation. Based on what I have learnt about CRPS and chronic pathological pain states I think we should be engaging with rehabilitation with the same attitude we take into stroke rehabilitation. I explain to patients with chronic pain that their brain has changed, that this change is a functional one but it manifests in some of the same ways that a minor stroke manifests. I emphasise the good news – that their brain is not damaged, which means that they can definitely retrain it. I explain pain (see[27] and[26] for reviews and links to a wider literature on explaining pain). I do not shirk the bad news – that the changes in the brain are difficult to reverse and require a great deal of practice.

Clinical quirk: *I remind patients, ad nauseum, that they will require **patience and persistence, courage and commitment**, all in large measure. It becomes a core theme of their training – patience and persistence, courage and commitment.*

Patience: *Take it one step at a time, do not exceed the training load because 'it feels good today'. I explain to patients that they will have really good days that leave them tempted to go beyond the planned load, but that this should be avoided. I justify this by emphasising the changes in sensitivity and that, if the brain is being overprotective of a body part because it is convinced that that body part needs protecting, then any increment in training that can be detected by this protective brain will evoke the very effective protective response – pain (along with other signs and symptoms).*

Persistence: *It will take a long time for GMI users to get there but the evidence and the biological rationale behind it strongly suggest that they will. I highlight the need to stay focused and to not flare-up, but not to freak out if they do because flare-ups are conceptualised as a protective strategy not a as a sign of reinjury.*

Courage: *I think that the complexity of pain means that there can be contributors and triggers that can only be confronted with a good dose of courage.*

Commitment: *One big challenge in the reality of a multidisciplinary and multipersonality medicosociolegal world is the continual appearance of people offering miraculous quick fixes, what I call the 'or-your-money-back' seduction. I take some time to convince patients that, on the basis of everything we know about the biology of chronic pain, and all the evidence we have on treating chronic pain, there is no quick fix. There is no magic pill or process. Instead, one must make the journey to recovery and be content along the way.*

Explaining graded motor imagery requires, in my view, a good understanding of it and more than likely, a conceptual endorsement of its underlying rationale. This issue has emerged in some clinical audits with which I have been involved[12]. Suffice here to say that two centres seem to have clearly worse results than the others. What is different about those centres? Are their patients more difficult than those at other centres? Were the staff just not trained well or are they inexperienced? Are the staff just losers?

Not surprisingly, the answer to all of these questions is a resounding 'No'. These two centres deservedly have a very good reputation and run highly evaluated multimodal evidence-based chronic pain rehabilitation. What is more the staff at those two centres are actually 'elite level clinicians' – they are highly qualified and experienced. They are, in some cases, world famous for their work in chronic pain. Yet their outcomes for graded motor imagery are not just 'no better' than the other centres, but, remarkably, they are *worse*. How do we explain that? I think the most likely explanation relates to the multimodal nature of intervention and the consequence that there are many explanatory models for the patient's pain. I suspect, although I have no hard data on this, that the conceptual model underpinning graded motor imagery might not be as well endorsed at those centres.

Clearly, finding out when something does not work is at least as important as finding out when it does. We need to do more research to disentangle all the contributors to outcomes, both good and bad. It is probably sufficient here though, to emphasise that the more complete the understanding and endorsement of the biological rationale of graded motor imagery the better. That is in part why we have written this book.

5.2 THE PRINCIPLE OF GRADED EXPOSURE AND RESPONSE PREVENTION

Let us return to the observation and subsequent research results that demonstrate that people with chronic limb pain can be aggravated by imagined movements. I interpret this to reflect sensitisation of the pain neurotag such that the motor command itself is sufficient to activate pain. Disinhibition would magnify this effect. Associative learning could also be a major contributor to this phenomenon – if movement hurts for long enough then the command to move will probably become sufficient to evoke pain. This association is difficult to unlearn because the pain still coincides with the movement, which confirms the association. One can see an immediate vicious cycle here. It is in my view not possible that the relationship is the other way around – that pain begins to evoke a movement response – because pain is the endpoint. To be the other way around would be a little like suggesting that Pavlov's dogs conditioned Pavlov – I cannot imagine them saying to each other, in dog-speak, 'Hey Ralph, watch this – every time I get some spit in my mouth, the guy with the beard goes and rings a bell'.

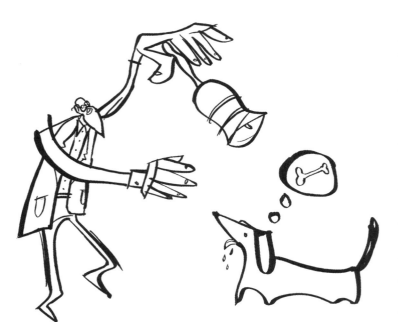

| *Figure 2.4* Remember Pavlov?

It makes sense to me that to avoid triggering a pain neurotag that is evoked by imagined movements, we need a stimulus that is less threatening than imagined movements. This principle is the linchpin of physical rehabilitation – if an activity is painful we deconstruct it slightly – we make it slower or shorter. We break it into components. We reduce the load or frequency or duration. Graded motor imagery is an extension of these principles to the neural substrate of movement and function. I have mentioned the distinction between implicit and explicit motor imagery. By moving from explicit to implicit I think we disengage the primary motor cortex.

I believe that disengaging the primary motor cortex has two excellent effects. First, it promotes inhibition (see section 2.1). This hypothesised effect is analogous to phrases used within the clinical community such as 'restoring laterality' and 'desmudging'. The second excellent effect is that it uncouples the hypothesised link between the primary motor cortex and the pain neurotag. It *dis*associates movement and pain. It seems that if we do this enough, we can then re-engage the primary motor cortex by explicit motor imagery in a way that does not evoke pain. Pavlov would be well pleased with this approach and I expect, its interpretation.

5.2.1 What if imagined movements do not cause pain? Where to start?

My approach to graded motor imagery has evolved over time and our outcome data across clinical centres with which I have been involved, reflect that evolution[17]. I think left/right judgements are a good place to start even if imagined movements are not painful because of the hypothesised effect of left/right judgements to promote intracortical inhibition and, therefore, the precision of motor neurotags. There are data to support this view – I compared the results of graded motor imagery to alternative forms of ungraded motor imagery in which imagined movements or mirror movements were undertaken first[24]. In short, the effects were fairly predictable – if imagined movements or mirror therapy were undertaken before left/right judgements, patients tended to get worse during those phases. When they were moved to left/right judgements, they tended to improve and if they *then* progressed to imagined movements they kept improving (Figure 2.5).

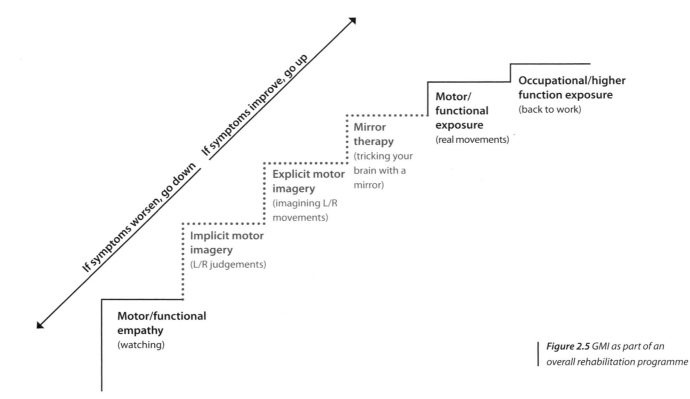

Figure 2.5 GMI as part of an overall rehabilitation programme

5.2.2 What if *implicit* motor imagery causes pain?

I have seen a smattering of people with CRPS and a couple of others with non-CRPS chronic severe pain whose pain worsened with implicit motor imagery, even after they have practiced it for a while and, presumably are no longer engaging their primary motor cortex. What on earth can be more conservative than implicit motor imagery? Our approach, which has anecdotally at least, seemed to be reasonably effective, is to use motor and functional empathy. This rather wishy-washy-sounding term is borne from the excellent work done by those clever Italians, on mirror neurones[41].

5.3 MIRROR NEURONES MAY OFFER SOME EXPLANATIONS

The possibility that our brains have a specialised capacity to imitate and that there are specific brain cells that do this job, was first reported by a group of Italian neuroscientists who were recording from individual brain cells in monkeys while the monkey ate some food. I have this account second hand, and it might just be an urban myth, but it makes for a fabulous story of serendipitous discovery.

By putting a monkey to sleep, inserting tiny electrodes into individual brain cells, then letting it wake up and go about its business, these neuroscientists were able to identify certain cells that were involved in hand function related to eating. Their electronic gadgets were able to convert the signal into a sound a bit like a morse code tapper, so they could 'listen' to the monkey's brain cells activating. Here is the cool part: the scientists stopped for lunch after a hard morning of neurophysiological drudgery, but forgot to turn off the equipment. Sitting in full view of the monkey, they broke out their calzone and pizza and were almost knocked off their Italian bottoms when they started to eat. Every time they took food to their mouth, they would hear the monkey's brain cells go beserk. If the scientists just moved a hand, nothing happened. But if they moved their hands to take food to their mouths, these brain cells would be activated, just as they were when the monkey did the same thing.

So, these lucky neuroscientists had discovered monkey brain cells that fire not only when the monkey takes food to its mouth, but also when the monkey watches another take food to its mouth. Mirror neurones. There is now a huge body of literature on mirror neurones in animals and humans. There are even journals dedicated to this system. Full coverage is beyond us here.

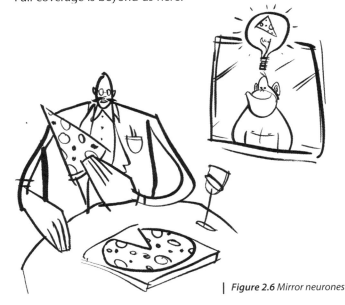

| *Figure 2.6 Mirror neurones*

However, it is a potentially important system to us because it implies that there are brain cells that can be activated when we watch someone else do something that we are not doing. That is, we might be unable or unwilling to do it because of pain, but if we watch someone else do it we can still access functionally-specific brain cells that are involved in doing it.

Before we go on however, we have to be clear that the whole idea of mirror neurones is not universally accepted – critics are not totally outnumbered by fans, at least in the cognitive neuroscience world. One critique which I find rather compelling has emerged as a result of the vast array of mirror neurones that have been uncovered almost all over the brain – and that is – 'If mirror neurones are everywhere, are we not just left with the perplexing problem of *How does the brain work?*' I don't claim for a second to have the smarts to discuss this at length but I do think we need to be aware that 'mirror neurone theory' is in many ways unfalsifiable, which leaves a reasonably large shadow over it. If you are interested in these thoughts here is a pretty digestible website that talks a great deal about it: www.talkingbrains.org.

Regardless of whether or not there is a particular type of neurone, or a particular system of mirror neurones, the discovery of this capacity of the human brain is enough to think more about whether it can be recruited within the context of rehabilitation. Let us go back to our proposed mechanism to further disengage the motor system in an effort to 'slip under the radar' of a sensitised pain neurotag and related disinhibition. When we watch someone else move we seem to provoke an automatic imitation of what they are doing. That is, simply perceiving someone else doing something or indeed touching something, or feeling something, evokes in us a very minor version of the same thing. For example, if we see a needle pricking the skin of someone else's hand, the excitability of brain cells that trigger movement of our own thumb are increased as though we too are trying to escape the needle[1]. So it seems reasonable to propose that, by watching other people walk we expose our brain to a very minor version of walking – almost certainly more minor than left/right judgements but nonetheless functionally specific. I suspect that watching someone else do something also primes the motor system in a manner that promotes desensitisation and inhibition. I have no evidence, but clinically our results have been good. Importantly practice, practice, practice.

5.3.1 Exploiting the mirror neurone system in rehabilitation

There are occasions when left/right judgements are unhelpful – I have seen patients whose pain worsens, others who feel nauseous, others who find it unbearably boring or unbearably difficult. I have had one patient who sneezed every time she started! One option in those scenarios is to think more conservatively and try motor or functional empathy. The principle is identical to that of graded motor imagery but simply involves watching people doing the movements or tasks to which we hope the patient progresses. To give you an idea of how this might look, Figure 2.7 describes Lucy Loo (not her real name), who presented with a 2 year history of CRPS, originally affecting one hand but by the time I saw her it also involved her face and leg.

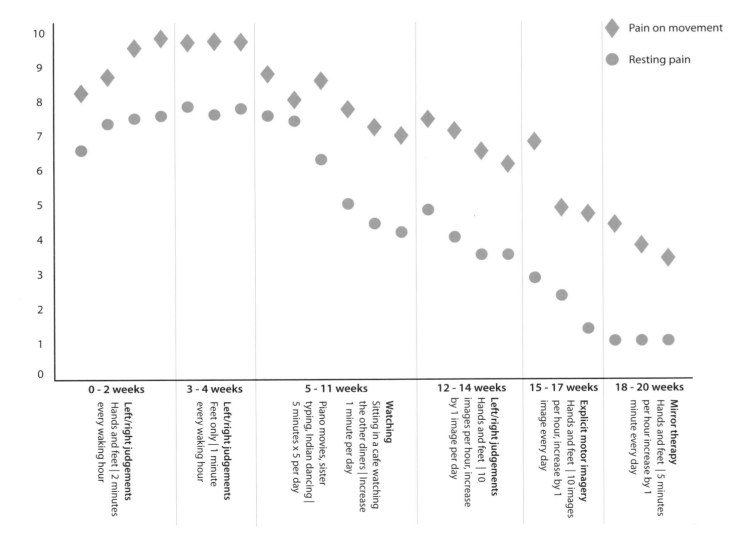

Figure 2.7 *Lucy Loo presented with marked CRPS affecting her arm, leg and face. We treated her with GMI for 2 minutes every waking hour for the first two weeks. Her pain worsened. You can see this by the slightly upward trajectory of the diamonds, which reflect pain on movement of her thumb, and the circles, which reflect pain at rest. We then reduced her training and worked on GMI of the feet instead. Two weeks later – no worse but really no better. We then did some motor empathy – we asked her to watch movies of people playing on the piano, watching her sister's hands as she typed at the computer, and to watch other movements. She clearly began to improve. We progressed that, spending more time and watching more functional activities, for 7 weeks. Then we tried GMI again and this time she responded. It took another 9 weeks to get through the GMI programme, but at 20 weeks after the initial appointment, Lucy started functional exposure. Six months later she had only a small amount of pain when she worked with her hands for half an hour or so. The trick with her? We had to get under the radar by abandoning GMI and starting instead with motor and functional empathy.*

Tim will describe the practical implementation of taking GMI 'backwards' to engage the mirroring capacity of the brain. We do not have hard empirical data on this extension of GMI, but we can base its implementation on principles that are proven in GMI and across rehabilitation in general.

- Some basic principles of motor/functional empathy: The idea is to have people watch, not in a vague absent minded way, but to really attend to the movements of other people.

- Watch in a fun place – watching people eat (from a distance and without being spotted!) can be great fun particularly if you are with someone else with a mischievous spirit!

- Watch with fun people.

- Movies are great – we use *Oscar Peterson: Music in the key of Oscar* for anyone who likes jazz music or used to play the piano; *Shine* for anyone who doesn't mind the piano.

- Always progress – do more today than yesterday but not much more.

5.4   EXPLICIT MOTOR IMAGERY

You will remember that the first stage of graded motor imagery is left/right judgements, or *implicit* motor imagery. The second stage of graded motor imagery is imagined movements, or *explicit* motor imagery. Earlier in this chapter, I discussed some of the useful differences between implicit motor imagery and explicit motor imagery and that

progressing from implicit to explicit was consistent with the principles of graded exposure. I also suggested that implicit motor imagery was a preferable place to start graded motor imagery because it clearly promotes inhibition or precision. I think that explicit motor imagery would still promote inhibition to some extent, but the key difference between explicit and implicit motor imagery is that the former will activate primary motor cortex (M1) cells and therefore, will activate the neurotags for movement.

The degree to which explicit motor imagery activates the neural mechanisms associated with actual movements is remarkable. The cortical activation is very similar, but movement-specific fluctuations are seen in lower motor neurones (those that reside in the front part of the spinal cord and directly activate muscle fibres) too. In fact, the muscles themselves often have movement-specific fluctuations in activity – very subtle – not enough to cause a movement but nonetheless visible to fairly run-of-the-mill recording equipment.

The extent to which explicit motor imagery mimics movements makes it an excellent training ground for those movements. That is, it is possible to almost fully recruit the command to move without running the risk of sensory feedback that will evoke pain. Explicit motor imagery is also very useful to engage the participant's brain with contextual and other factors that may be contributing to the difficulty with some movements or behaviours. Can those factors really make a difference? Well consider these two factors:

A. The lower motor neurone gets about 50% of its projections from areas *other than* the primary motor cortex; movements are organised functionally in the motor cortex, not anatomically. This means that there are other brain areas that can directly modulate activity of the neurones that supply muscles, which means that they directly modulate activity of muscles.

B. The motor cortex is organised functionally, not by muscles. This is a very important consideration because it means that the one brain cell might contribute to the neurotag of elbow flexion and the neurotag of wrist deviation because it is part of the neurotag of drinking a beer.

By undertaking explicit motor imagery with a programme such as Recognise, it is possible to directly train the range of movements we are likely to encounter in life by using the context images rather than the vanilla images. There is another advantage too – in much the same way that observing another person doing something runs the neural hardware for doing the same task in us, explicit motor imagery does this in the sensory domain as well as in the motor domain. So, if we imagine using a hammer, then not only do we run the neurotag of using a hammer, we also send messages that 'prime' the sensory brain cells to 'expect' sensory input in line with using a hammer. The sensory brain cells that would be activated while using a hammer include those that register compression of the skin on the palm of the hand and fingers, elbow movement, the sound of the hammer hitting the nail etc etc. This by-product of imagined movements seems to me to be an excellent way to train inhibition or precision within the sensory system in much the same way that left/right judgements train precision within the motor system.

5.4.1 A useful take-home message regarding explicit motor imagery

Try progressing the patient from vanilla to context images as soon as you can. Monitor their symptoms and signs – if vanilla images are fine but context images aggravate them, you can be reasonably sure that the context is the aggravator – now you have to find which of the images are sufficiently threatening to be activating the pain neurotag. In my experience, patients will be able to identify themselves which of the images they saw makes them feel a bit edgy or fearful. If not, you could try asking them 'Did any of those images show an activity that would make your pain worse?'

When you find the culprit images, you may need to directly de-threaten them, or break them down to sufficiently non-threatening components as to not increase pain (or other signs or symptoms). Here is a patient example.

Mrs F was progressing well from implicit motor imagery using vanilla images, then to explicit motor imagery using context images. Her pain however, would increase during explicit imagery on about half her training sessions. Using the process outlined above, we identified one image in particular that was a likely culprit – a picture of a hand pruning the roses. So we broke that task down, just as we would if we were doing the actual task:

Step 1: Mrs F would imagine picking up the snippers and putting them back again.

Step 2: Imagine gently squeezing the snippers and relaxing.

Step 3: Imagine a cool breeze on her face and then squeeze the snippers hard.

Step 4: Imagine a cool breeze on her face, her favourite music playing in the background, and snipping off a branch. For this component she concentrated on the feel of the breeze, then the music, then the visual appearance of the rose bush, positioning the snippers, watching the blades slowly come together.

This whole process took about 10 minutes. She was able to imagine pruning without it increasing her pain. She went back to context Recognise exercises, without an increase in symptoms, and progressed through her graded motor imagery programme.

5.5 MIRROR THERAPY

The final component of graded motor imagery before progressing onto functional exposure, is mirror therapy. You will remember from earlier in this chapter that there is good evidence that the order of graded motor imagery – implicit motor imagery, explicit motor imagery, mirror therapy – seems to be important[24]. In fact, the research that has been undertaken so far does not clearly show the contribution of mirror therapy to graded motor imagery – our experimental designs stopped short of fully interrogating this. However, there is a large amount of literature now available on mirror therapy – we wrote what we think is an even-handed review a few years ago, but not much has changed since[31].

Rather than rewrite it all here, it is fair to say that mirror therapy on its own, does not have a measurable advantage over explicit motor imagery as a way of treating chronic painful disorders (although it probably does for stroke rehabilitation – a whole other kettle of fish and one well worth writing a book on – just not this book!) Our own research has not ruled out the possibility that the treatment effects of graded motor imagery would be similar (or indeed better) if the mirror therapy component was replaced with further explicit motor imagery, or was skipped and treatment was progressed straight to functional movements. There are three caveats here though:

A. There is a good biology-based argument to not skip mirror therapy: by providing visual feedback of the healthy limb, a limb that looks well, moves well and is fully endorsed by the brain, mirror therapy provides a smaller jump in terms of threatening load, from explicit motor imagery to functional exposure. In my own experience, skipping this jump can incur such a large progression that the patient 'falls off' the rehabilitation ladder.

B. I have never had a patient get immediate and 'fantastic' pain relief from motor imagery, but I have had many who get it from mirror therapy. Not quite in the style shown by Dr House, nor even described by Ramachandran, but significant enough for them to carry a mirror box around with them instead of a packet of paracetamol (acetaminophen).

C. There are very capable and clever clinicians who swear by mirror therapy. I have not seen the results that they describe, but I know they are top-notch clinicians and very fine people. This plants a whispering in my brain that mirror therapy can be more effective on its own than I have found it to be. Time will tell – I look forward to seeing high-quality clinical trials that really test mirror therapy in people with chronic pain.

Mirror therapy has one clear advantage over motor imagery – it is far more engaging and novel and fun. This is of critical importance because perhaps the biggest challenge facing the clinician and the patient is sustaining motivation and engagement. Mirror therapy is very useful in this regard. The general principle of mirror therapy is to perform movements with both hands but look at the reflected image of the good hand, rather than look at the bad hand. This limits somewhat the repertoire of movements that can be used – it is probably not very helpful to try writing with both hands! There are other twists and turns that can be manipulated with mirror therapy – Tim will discuss that in the next chapter. The key is to engage with mirror therapy within a strong clinical reasoning model, which David discusses in the introductory chapter. Without strong clinical reasoning, mirror therapy, indeed graded motor imagery could well be as effective as a boat without a rudder.

6. DOES GRADED MOTOR IMAGERY WORK?

There are two randomised controlled trials[1], a randomised comparative clinical trial[24], which together included 84 patients, and two systematic reviews[3]. We also have very tight observational data from 201 *consecutive* and 59 near consecutive* CRPS or phantom limb pain patients who undertook rehabilitation that included but was not limited to, graded motor imagery and was firmly based on the same underlying conceptual paradigm. Finally, we have data from another 45 near consecutive CRPS patients who undertook graded motor imagery within centres who delivered multimodal treatments with differing underlying conceptual paradigms.

At the highest level of evidence (systematic reviews), graded motor imagery is considered effective for reducing pain and disability in people with acute and chronic CRPS or phantom limb pain. The 305-patient audit data are remarkably consistent with the clinical trials, with the exception of the data from the two centres mentioned above. I have suggested that their results may be hampered by multiple explanatory models or incomplete endorsement of the principles underpinning graded motor imagery.

* Being consecutive is important because it shows that we did not 'cherry pick' the patients who we thought, for some reason or another and possibly even unconsciously, would do better. Always look for this in observational studies – if it is called a convenience sample, the risk of bias is much greater.

Of course, we need to hold up the mirror and ask whether their audit data might just be better collected or less biased than the data from the other centres. Perhaps because they are so famous for their treatment of CRPS, they just see patients who are worse off and less likely to respond. Maybe it is a quirky blip in the data. We don't know at this stage but it is certainly worth thinking about.

At this stage, there are no empirical data that I know about from people who have other types of pain – that is, not CRPS or phantom limb pain. There are anecdotal data but case studies tend to be overly positive about a treatment – who wants to write up a patient for whom treatment was not effective? What editor really wants to publish it? Clearly we need more research. I can hear Dave groan at this, but it does not mean that we need to sit back and wait for those academic types to do a randomised controlled trial (RCT). RCTs are very time consuming and expensive – a good one will cost over a million dollars – and they are not the only type of evidence worth having, although they are almost certainly the best. Instead, coalface clinicians can undertake their own research in exactly the same way we have, by properly auditing their data. It really just comes down to accurate and standardised reporting and including consecutive patients. One can develop a very simple data collection tool that has a few fields to tell you about the patient, the key variables of interest (I think pain and disability are the best) and standardised time points – pre, 6 weeks, 6 months. The only mildly tricky part is getting the 6 month data – we phone people. We phone them for 6 week data if they have been discharged. The key thing

is to make sure consecutive patients are included. If the data are from consecutive patients and they suggest the outcomes are good, then we use that to convince someone to fund an RCT. That clinicians do not seem to get involved in this process is just as frustrating to me as the erroneous conclusion held by many scientists, that a treatment does not work if there is no evidence to prove it.

In summary: As far as the evidence tells us, graded motor imagery is one of the best treatments for CRPS and PLP, but its effectiveness probably depends on many factors. Graded motor imagery may or may not be effective for other pain states – we just do not know yet. Clinicians can directly contribute to the evidence by being diligent collectors of information.

7.   CONCLUDING REMARKS FOR THIS CHAPTER

The purpose of this chapter is to provide the background, theoretical basis and current state of the evidence concerning graded motor imagery. I have tried to convey what are in places quite complicated biological processes in a manner that is accurate but not too overwhelming. The interested reader could go directly to the scientific articles to learn more. All of the articles written by my research group are freely available as PDFs at: www.bodyinmind.org, where there are also slideshows on training the brain and some other resources. I have several objectives that I hope have been achieved. I hope the reader understands:

A. That there is over a decade of clinical research behind graded motor imagery, and several decades of more fundamental research behind that.

B. That there are sensible interpretations of how people perform on left/right judgements, but these interpretations should be considered general rules, not 'hard and fast' rules.

C. That there is a sensible biological explanation for why graded motor imagery might work.

D. That there is strong but not yet irrefutable, evidence that graded motor imagery reduces pain and disability in people with CRPS or phantom limb pain.

E. That it is important to *understand* graded motor imagery and to apply it within a framework that embraces all the excellent things we know about rehabilitation (this is covered better in following chapters).

F. That there is a solid argument to suggest that the application of graded motor imagery will extend well beyond the treatment of people with CRPS or phantom limb pain. The research to determine if this is true is still underway.

G. Clinicians can contribute to our understanding of graded motor imagery by undertaking precise audits.

REFERENCES

1. Avenanti A, Bueti D, Galati G, et al. Transcranial magnetic stimulation highlights the sensorimotor side of empathy for pain. Nat Neurosci 2005;8:955-60.

2. Butler D, Moseley GL. *Explain Pain*. Adelaide: Noigroup Publications, 2003.

3. Daly AE, Bialocerkowski AE. Does evidence support physiotherapy management of adult Complex Regional Pain Syndrome Type One? A systematic review. Eur J Pain 2009;13:339-53.

4. Decety J. Do imagined and executed actions share the same neural substrate? Cognitive Brain Research 1996;3:87-93.

5. Decety J. The neurophysiological basis of motor imagery. Behav Brain Res 1996;77:45-52.

6. Flor H, Braun C, Elbert T, et al. Extensive reorganization of primary somatosensory cortex in chronic back pain patients. Neurosci Lett 1997;224:5-8.

7. Flor H, Elbert T, Knecht S, et al. Phantom-limb pain as a perceptual correlate of cortical reorganization following arm amputation. Nature 1995;375:482-4.

8. Flor H, Nikolajsen L, Jensen TS. Phantom limb pain: a case of maladaptive CNS plasticity? Nat Rev Neurosci 2006;7:873-81.

9. Gustin SM, Wrigley PJ, Gandevia SC, et al. Movement imagery increases pain in people with neuropathic pain following complete thoracic spinal cord injury. Pain 2008;137:237-44.

10. Harris AJ. Cortical origin of pathological pain. Lancet 1999;354:1464-6.

11. Hudson ML, McCormick K, Zalucki N, et al. Expectation of pain replicates the effect of pain in a hand laterality recognition task: Bias in information processing toward the painful side? Eur J Pain 2006;10:219-24.

12. Johnson S, Hall J, Draper M, et al. Using graded motor imagery for complex regional pain syndrome in clinical practice: Failure to improve pain. European Journal of Pain 2011.

13. Lotze M, Moseley GL. Role of distorted body image in pain. Curr Rheumatol Rep 2007;9:488-96.

14. Maihofner C, Handwerker HO, Neundorfer B, et al. Patterns of cortical reorganization in complex regional pain syndrome. Neurology 2003;61:1707-15.

15. Melzack R. Phantom limbs and the concept of a neuromatrix. Trends Neurosci 1990;13:88-92.

16. Melzack R, Israel R, Lacroix R, et al. Phantom limbs in people with congenital limb deficiency or amputation in early childhood. Brain 1997;120:1603-20.

17. Moseley G. Rehabilitation of complex regional pain syndrome. In Mogil J ed. World Congress on Pain. Montreal, Canada: IASP Press, 2010:125-36.

18. Moseley G, Acerra N. Complex Regional Pain Syndrome is associated with distorted body image of the affected part. J Neurol Sci 2005;238:S501-S.

19. Moseley GL. Distorted body image in complex regional pain syndrome. Neurology 2005;65:773-.

20. Moseley GL. Graded motor imagery for pathologic pain - A randomized controlled trial. Neurology 2006;67:2129-34.

21. Moseley GL. Graded motor imagery is effective for long-standing complex regional pain syndrome: a randomised controlled trial. Pain 2004;108:192-8.

22. Moseley GL. I can't find it! Distorted body image and tactile dysfunction in patients with chronic back pain. Pain 2008;140:239-43.

23. Moseley GL. Imagined movements cause pain and swelling in a patient with complex regional pain syndrome. Neurology 2004;62:1644.

24. Moseley GL. Is successful rehabilitation of complex regional pain syndrome due to sustained attention to the affected limb? A randomised clinical trial. Pain 2005;114:54-61.

25. Moseley GL. Making sense of S1 mania - are things really that simple? In Gifford L ed. Topical Issues in Pain Volume 5. Falmouth: CNS Press, 2006:321-40.

26. Moseley GL. A pain neuromatrix approach to patients with chronic pain. Man Ther 2003;8:130-40.

27. Moseley GL. Reconceptualising pain according to its underlying biology. Physical Therapy Reviews 2007;12:169-78.

28. Moseley GL. Why do people with complex regional pain syndrome take longer to recognize their affected hand? Neurology 2004;62:2182-6.

29. Moseley GL, Birklein F, van Hilten BJ, et al. Imagined movements in CRPS - reply to Hall et al. Arthritis & Rheumatism-Arthritis Care & Research 2009;61:140-1.

30. Moseley GL, Gallace A, Spence C. Bodily illusions in health and disease: physiological and clinical perspectives and the concept of a cortical body matrix. Neurosci Biobehav Rev 2012: 36:34-46.

31. Moseley GL, Gallace A, Spence C. Is mirror therapy all it is cracked up to be? Current evidence and future directions. Pain 2008;138:7-10.

32. Moseley GL, Gallace A, Spence C. Space-based, but not arm-based, shift in tactile processing in complex regional pain syndrome and its relationship to cooling of the affected limb. Brain 2009;132:3142-51.

33. Moseley GL, Gandevia SC. Re: Sensory-motor incongruence and reports of 'pain', by G. L. Moseley and S. C. Gandevia. Rheumatology 2005;44 : 1083-1085: Reply. Rheumatology 2006;45:645-.

34. Moseley GL, Gandevia SC. Sensory-motor incongruence and reports of 'pain'. Rheumatology 2005;44:1083-5.

35. Moseley GL, Schweinhardt P, Wise R, et al. Virtual, imagined and mirror movements - a novel approach to complex regional pain syndrome (CRPS1). European Federation of IASP Chapters Triennial Conference. Prague, Czech Republic, 2003: Abstract 686T p422.

36. Moseley GL, Sim DF, Henry ML, et al. Experimental hand pain delays recognition of the contralateral hand - evidence that acute and chronic pain have opposite effects on information processing? Cog Brain Res 2005;25:188-94.

37. Moseley GL, Zalucki N, Birklein F, et al. Thinking about movement hurts: The effect of motor imagery on pain and swelling in people with chronic arm pain. Arthritis Care Res 2008;59:623-31.

38. Moseley HL, Gallagher L, Gallace A. Neglect-like tactile dysfunction in chronic back pain. Neurology 2012 (in press).

39. Parsons LM. Integrating cognitive psychology, neurology and neuroimaging. Acta Psychol (Amst) 2001;107:155-81.

40. Ramachandran VS, Blakeslee S. Phantoms in the brain. First ed. New York: William Morrow, 1998.

41. Rizzolatti G, Craighero L. The mirror-neuron system. Annu Rev
    Neurosci 2004;27:169-92.

42. Schwoebel J, Friedman R, Duda N, et al. Pain and the body
    schema: evidence for peripheral effects on mental
    representations of movement. Brain 2001;124:2098-104.

43. Tracey I. Functional connectivity and pain: How effectively
    connected is your brain? Pain 2005;116:173-4.

44. Wand BM, Parkitny L, O'Connell NE, et al. Cortical changes
    in chronic low back pain: Current state of the art and
    implications for clinical practice. Man Ther 2011;16:15-20.

45. Woolf CJ, Salter M. Plasticity and pain: the role of the dorsal
    horn. In McMahon SB, Koltzenburg M eds. *Textbook of
    Pain.* 5th ed. London: Elsevier, 2006:91-107.

NOTES

Treatment through Graded Motor Imagery
Timothy B. Beames

1. INTRODUCTION

Graded motor imagery (GMI) is a treatment process aimed at helping people with persistent and complex pain states. The treatment has been used successfully for people with complex regional pain syndrome, phantom limb pain and pain following brachial plexus injury. We believe that it may be an important approach for many other pain problems as well. I am a clinician treating people with complex pain states and I also teach these imagery strategies to other clinicians. It is an exciting time for GMI, reflected by the interest shown by my patients, the clinicians who attend the courses and the expanding evidence base. I'm eternally indebted to my patients and colleagues for what they have taught me and hope to share some of that knowledge in this chapter.

GMI is essentially a brain-based treatment, targeting the activation of different brain regions in a graded manner. Treatment consists of three different components that include the rehabilitation of left/right discrimination of the affected area, motor imagery rehearsal and mirror therapy. It incorporates the use of computers, magazines, flash cards, mirrors and imagination. It is also hard work.

This chapter is aimed at helping clinicians and patients (the users) to make the best decisions in GMI. This means knowing when to choose the most appropriate approaches within GMI, being able to adapt the approaches to suit the user and to make best informed decisions about when to move forwards, backwards or sideways with their treatment.

In this chapter there are dialogues between patients, therapists and me. Following these dialogues there is a small amount of information guiding the user towards best practice from current research and our experience. The aim of this is to provide flexible and creative routes to tackle individual problems. Let's first take a look at the graded part of GMI.

GMI
hand
book

2. THE GRADED PART OF GMI

2.1 GRADED EXPOSURE

Graded motor imagery fits broadly under a process called graded exposure – a widely used approach to treating pain and movement problems. It is sometimes referred to as 'pacing', although we believe it is much more than this. The approach has been successfully used in rehabilitation for tissue injuries, complex pain problems and phobia management. The classic literature on this subject includes Vlaeyen[15] and Leeuw[4]. Consider a sportsman who has damaged his knee – he doesn't go straight back to competition. He goes through a progression of rehabilitation, usually doing a little bit more than the day before (but not always). This will include a breakdown of specific tasks such as strengthening and stretching exercises and involves training in different contexts such as in the gym or on the field. In relation to GMI we use similar principles but with a focus on brain training.

Graded exposure requires appropriate education regarding pain and activity, drawing up goals to work towards, possibly with the use of a fear hierarchy which I will discuss later (see Figure 3.9), and the gradual exposure to the activities that have become more limited due to pain. This gradual exposure to activities will take on board contextual challenges such as changes in emotion or the environment. For example, in a GMI approach, practicing left/right discrimination exercises on a computer when you are stressed, when you are happy, when you are at work, or in the safety of your home can be graded according to the degree of challenge each situation offers for you.

Repeating and gradually 'exposing' the activity in an appropriate way and changing the contextual challenges often allows a reduction in pain and a gradual improvement in activity. This is likely to be due to the brain becoming happier and less threatened by these activities. The brain has a huge ability to be flexible and creative in performing the same tasks. It is this flexibility and creativity that we are aiming to give back to it. Graded exposure is also discussed in David's chapter and in 'Explain Pain'[2].

2.2 TWO WAYS OF GRADING IN GMI

GMI is graded in two ways. Firstly, it is a sequential process where a reasonable ability in left/right discrimination is required before moving to the next step of imagining movement and then mirror therapy[8]. GMI appears to be most effective when kept in this order (Figure 3.1). This means that someone with persistent pain will benefit most (in terms of a reduction in pain and improvement in function that is maintained) when trained in left/right discrimination prior to practicing explicit motor imagery and will be more likely to improve using mirrors in treatment after being trained in left/right discrimination and motor imagery[10].

We believe that each stage allows an increase in the firing of the brain regions involved in the desired activity and aims to avoid setting off the pain neurotag in the brain. Neurotags are essentially a collection of brain areas firing together to produce a pain experience and they are described in more detail in Lorimer and David's chapters or in *'Explain Pain'*. I will discuss each of the three stages in turn later in the chapter. Secondly, grading can also be carried out within each of the three stages, by altering the amount and kind of activity. It is this part of the grading that we will focus on in this chapter.

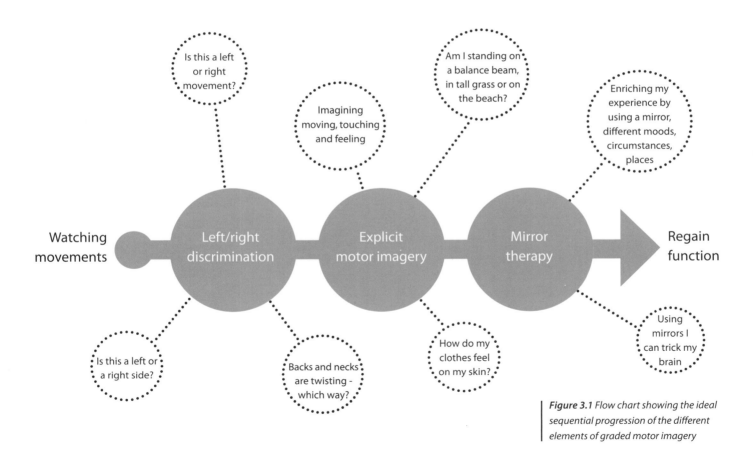

GMI hand book

Figure 3.1 Flow chart showing the ideal sequential progression of the different elements of graded motor imagery

2.3 BASELINES AND FLARE-UPS

The 'graded' part of graded motor imagery is so important
and we believe that users may need to accept the
importance of this simple sounding strategy first. To begin
graded activity a *baseline* level of activity (or thinking of an
activity) needs to be worked out first. Then the amount of
activity needs to be increased over time. That sounds very
simple! The more activity that can be accomplished without
creating a *flare-up* (for example, something that wipes you
out for a day or makes you reach for the drugs) progressively
disassociates that activity from pain, so your brain is
relearning. The 'twin peaks' model in David's next chapter
takes these issues further and I'll discuss baselines and flare-
ups when I present patients' stories later in the chapter.

Lorimer talks about the need to be patient and persistent.
Essentially it's important to take treatment one step at a
time and not exceed the predetermined training load. It
takes time for the sensitivity to improve and for the brain to
become happy with each change. Therefore, it is important
to allow some time and repetition of activities within the
safe baseline and avoid flare-ups that will maintain or
increase sensitivity of the pain neurotag. The brain probably
needs to experience success in each activity a number of
times and in many different contexts.

3. THE THREE STAGES OF GMI

The next section goes through each part of the graded
motor imagery process. It provides examples of the
principles of graded exposure to guide the progression of
rehabilitation. The first part looks at left/right discrimination
– implicit (unconscious) motor imagery – and shows how
to take a step back when just imagining moving is painful.
Following this there is a section on explicit motor imagery
or the act of consciously imagining movements. The
process is concluded with the use of mirrors.

4. LEFT/RIGHT DISCRIMINATION (IMPLICIT MOTOR IMAGERY)

4.1 INTRODUCTION AND DEFINITION

The left/right discrimination (laterality) tasks are designed to assess how easily you can judge if the image you are looking at is a left or right body part (see Figure 3.2) or in the case of the spine (Figure 3.3), whether that person is turning to the left or to the right. We are interested in collecting information about the accuracy and the speed of the response.

The task is likely to link to the unconscious brain representation of a person's body part and/or movement of it. Lorimer has written extensively on the neuroscience of left/right judgement tasks in the previous chapter.

An important aspect of the test is that it is performed unconsciously (relatively). This means that it should be done as quickly as possible, almost as though you were guessing. Essentially there will be less activation of movement areas in the brain and you will access deep movement planning areas by performing it in this way.

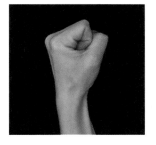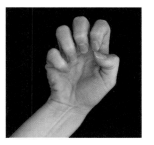

Figure 3.2 Vanilla images (with a plain background) of hands in different positions. Are these images of left or right hands?

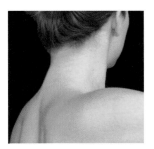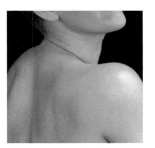

Figure 3.3 Vanilla images of necks in different positions. Is this person turning to the left or to the right?

4.2   TOOLS TO ASSESS AND TREAT LEFT/RIGHT DISCRIMINATION CHANGES

4.2.1 Computer programmes

The best way to test left right discrimination abilities is to use the online Recognise programme www.noigroup.com/recognise. Here, images of body parts are programmed to come up on a computer screen and you can select the body part, number of images, the amount of time the image is held on the screen and the degree of difficulty of the image. You can even put your own images on the screen. Tom discusses the use of this programme step by step in chapter 5 and I discuss training via the programme in section 4.3 below. The programme also provides a way of treating any changes in discrimination abilities and it provides a record so that progress can be monitored. A Recognise App is also available and Tom also discusses this in chapter 5.

4.2.2 Magazine Therapy

Not everyone has access to a computer. Magazines can be used to provide a crude guide to assess left/right discrimination abilities and they can also be used for training. It certainly offers a nice contextual exercise, gets you away from the computer for a bit and second hand shops usually have heaps of old magazines for very cheap.

Take a magazine and a pen and go through the magazine circling the targeted part – so a right hand if yours is a right hand problem or a person turning to the left if you are dealing with a neck problem when you turn to the left (Figure 3.4). We suggest that you use a variety of magazines – ones you like and even some you don't like – it all makes for good brain exercise. You may become aware of some idea of a left/right discrimination problem while using magazines, but it will be best to quantify any problem by using the online Recognise programme. There is some recent evidence suggesting that magazine exercises can be made more difficult by rotating the magazine[16]. The speed and accuracy of left/right discrimination will be best at 0 degrees and increasingly slower and less accurate at 90, 270 and 180 degrees (Figure 3.5).

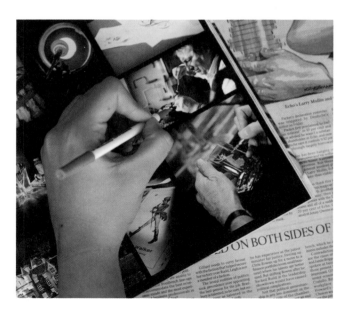

Figure 3.4 Use of a magazine for left/ right discrimination training. In this case, all the right hands are identified and circled.

One important thing about left/right discrimination exercises is that you don't get too involved in the images. The decision of left or right has to be something of an unconscious guess. It might be best not to choose pictures that you find too interesting!

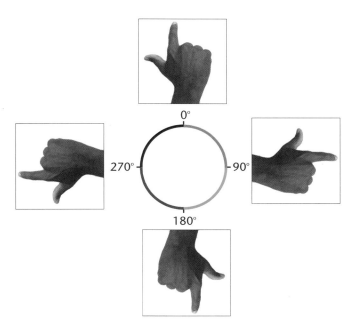

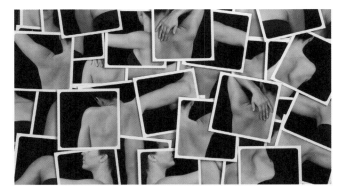

4.2.3 Flash Cards

Flash cards are a set of 48 cards, just a little larger than a pack of cards. They have 24 images of a body part and the reverse image giving a total of 48 images (Figure 3.6). Similar to the magazines, there are obvious limitations for assessment but they can provide some indication of accuracy. Their major role is in treatment once a left/right discrimination issue has been identified. One advantage of the flash cards is that they can be used in different contexts, for example in the bus or at work. The major challenge using flash cards is to keep the task as unconscious as possible, because the longer it takes the more likely the task will be a conscious one and therefore falls into the realms of explicit motor imagery or consciously imagining movement.

Figure 3.5 The speed and accuracy of left/right discrimination will be best at 0 degrees and increasingly slower and less accurate at 90, 270 and 180 degrees.

Figure 3.6 Flash cards are a set of 24 images and reversed images of a body part.

The simplest way to start is to draw an 'R' and 'L' on paper in front of you and then to go through the cards, placing left sided ones on the 'L' and right on the 'R' (Figure 3.7).

There are a number of other ways to assess and treat using flash cards. For example, you could write an 'R' or 'L' on the back of the cards and get someone (with good left right discrimination) to check yours.

The flash cards produced by NOI include information about some games which could be used as treatment such as left/right noughts and crosses (Figure 3.8). Once again, try to make the left/right decisions as rapidly as possible. These cards are available for the hands, feet, backs and necks. Of course, it would not be difficult to make your own cards using your own hands if you are a patient.

Flash cards are also one method to help you work out a fear hierarchy of specific movements. Place them in order of expected pain, discomfort or difficulty from least to most (or in 3 or 4 separate piles as in Figure 3.9). As a way of grading the exercises, the user could work at exercises from the least threatening to the most threatening cards. This grading could be used for both stage 1 and stage 2 of GMI. There is further discussion on the use of cards in the explicit motor imagery section later in the chapter.

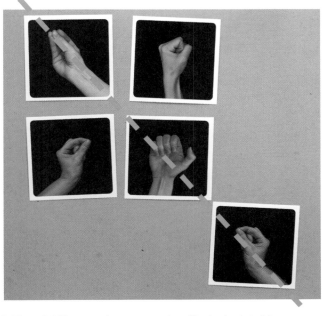

Figure 3.8 *Many popular games can be utilised as brain training excercises – for example, link lefts or rights instead of noughts and crosses in 'Tic-tac-toe'. Try also 'Snap' and 'Fish'. The brochure accompanying the flash card pack has other suggestions.*

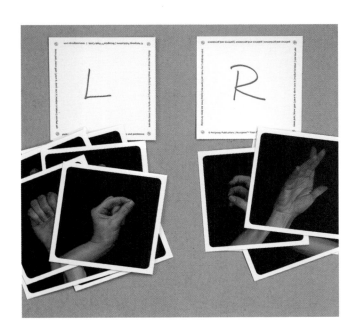

| **Figure 3.7** *Assessing left/right discrimination using flash cards*

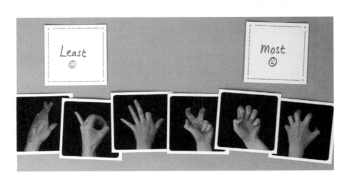

| **Figure 3.9** *Working out a fear hierarchy using flash cards.*

GMI
hand
book

4.3   RECOGNISE ONLINE

4.3.1 Familiarising yourself with the process and getting started

The following discussion involves use of the online Recognise programme.

As mentioned above, the left/right discrimination task involves guessing whether you are looking at either a right or left body part or posture. I am saying it is a guess but the brain works so quickly to recognise whether it is a left or right body part (or movement) that you won't be conscious that you've done it. This may mean that it feels like you are just guessing!

When beginning the online assessment it may be appropriate to familiarise yourself with the task by performing the test for another body part or region first, particularly when the body part that you want to treat is very sensitive. Let's discuss this via the example of a patient, Jane.

Jane, 38, has complex regional pain syndrome 1 of the left foot and leg, which came on following an injury. She has had this problem for 6 years and experiences constant, severe pain. This has led to the need for her to use a wheelchair to move around the house. Despite this she continues to run her own small craft business making cards from her home. At the time of her initial assessment she was experiencing almost daily flare-ups. She achieves some pain relief through the administration of intravenous ketamine infusions at her local hospital.

I assessed Jane's left/right discrimination. It was reasoned that starting with her hands would be better than beginning with her feet. This was in order to avoid potential adverse responses due to the sensitivity of her pain neurotag and also to give her some understanding of what to expect of the task.

Jane was given some prior instruction of what the program would display and the keys on the keyboard that she needed to press that identify left and right body parts. She was also asked not to take too long thinking about the process or moving her body to match the image displayed.

To begin with Jane was shown 20 images of vanilla hands and each image was displayed for a maximum of 20 seconds. This would be considered a moderate number of images and a long period of time for the images to be shown but from my history taking I reasoned that Jane's foot problem was very sensitive. The accuracy and speed results are shown below in graphs from Recognise (Figures 3.10 and 3.11).

The results show the accuracy (Figure 3.10) in terms of the percentage of correct guesses and the response time (Figure 3.11). There is an improvement in both the accuracy and response times for Jane following repetition of the task over the first few days. The initial response times are slow and therefore likely to indicate that the process is very much conscious. However, they quickly improve. This may be a learning effect but may also be due to prompts given to Jane to keep the test unconscious.

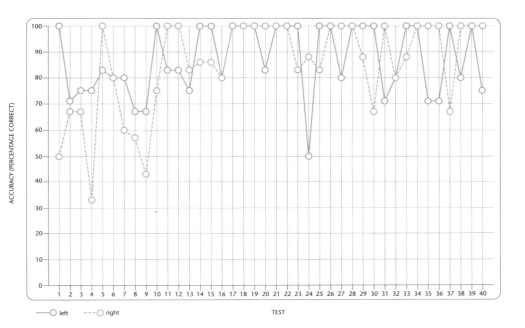

ACCURACY (PERCENTAGE CORRECT)

TEST

○— left   ---○ right

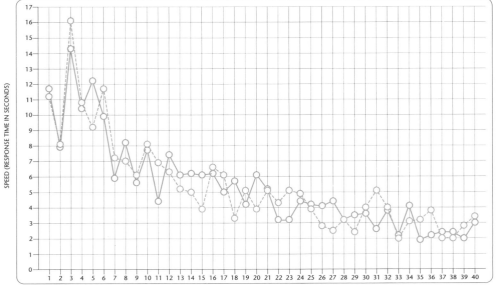

SPEED (RESPONSE TIME IN SECONDS)

TEST

○— left   ---○ right

Figure 3.10 *Left/right accuracy scores for Jane. Tests 1-4 were familiarising tests for the hand and the rest of the tests are for the feet. Note the 'fadeout' for the left foot in test 24 and how she achieves more accurate scores for the right (good) foot than the left. This graph shows data collected over 13 days. Orange = LHS accuracy, green = RHS accuracy.*

Figure 3.11 *Initial assessment of response time (seconds) of Jane's left/right discrimination in hands and feet. Tests 1-4 are familiarising tests for hands. Tests 5-39 are for feet. While improvement over time is clearly shown, there is no evidence of any difference between left and right response times. These tests show data collected over 13 days. Orange = LHS response times. Green = RHS response times.*

GMI
hand
book

4.3.2 Training effects of Recognise

Jane has worked hard. In figures 3.10 and 3.11, it is clear that Jane's left/right discrimination scores, especially response times, have improved over 13 days. Let's take a look at what happened some months later where the results are shown in figures 3.12 and 3.13. These are results that the user should be aiming for. Here Jane has progressed onto different contexts of images. It also shows that she has included her hands and mixed up the context of the test so as not to repeat the same one each time. (What is not shown is that she has also increased the number of images and reduced the time that they are shown, following a graded exposure approach).

These results show that Jane's left/right discrimination for feet has improved and that the accuracy is above 92% and that all response times for the feet are below 1.3 seconds and fall well within what we now consider to be normal values following training. It also demonstrates that these values are reasonably stable and do not fluctuate greatly from day to day or over several weeks. Interestingly Jane is one of a number of people who struggle with their left and right with dyslexia. Her improvements in left/right discrimination tasks were mimicked by improvements in other tasks such as map reading skills! With results like this it is time for Jane to move onto explicit motor imagery (section 5).

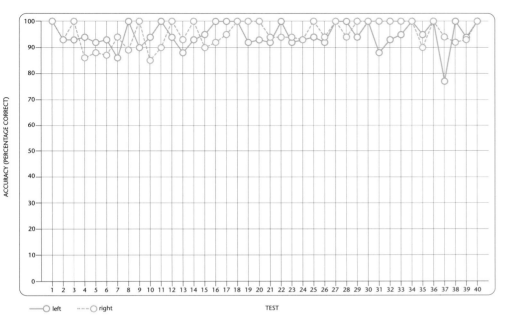

Figure 3.12 *Jane's Recognise left/right discrimination results following practice. The results show that the accuracy is above 92%. The responses are reasonably equal from side to side. This data was collected over 20 days, 9 months after the initial assessment data shown in Figure 3.10. Orange = LHS accuracy, green = RHS accuracy.*

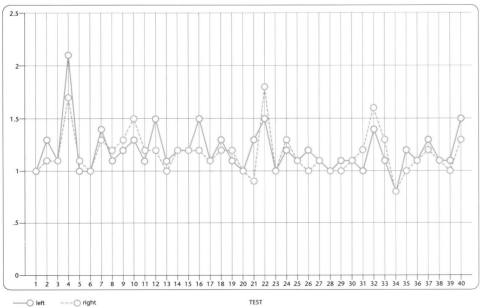

Figure 3.13 *Jane's Recognise left/right response times following practice. The results show that the response times for the feet average around 1.3 seconds. The responses are reasonably equal from side to side. This data was collected over 20 days, 9 months after the initial assessment data shown in Figure 3.11. Orange = LHS response time, green= RHS response time.*

GMI
hand
book

4.3.3 What is normal?

We have suggested that Jane's results are normal. For the past 2 years, we have been researching left/right discrimination and among other things, have tried to get a sense of what are 'normal' responses. It is very easy to argue about what normal is, and here we are offering guidelines based on our research. Sarah Wallwork[16] sampled 1,749 people in an online study where she looked at hand and neck left/right discrimination speed and accuracy. Jane Bowering[1] used the same methodology to obtain data that allows us to provide some guidance about what are normal accuracy and response times for the low back.

Our broad suggestions for normal responses to a left/right discrimination test are:

- Accuracy of 80% and above, but see Figure 3.14A-E for some variations.

- A speed of 1.6 seconds +/- 0.5 sec appears quite normal for necks and backs. Hands and feet are a little slower with an average speed of 2 seconds +/- 0.5 sec. We do not have data at the time of publishing for other body parts, so we suggest that around 2 seconds is quite normal for the limbs.

- Accuracies and response times should be reasonably equal left and right.

- The patient results should be quite stable, so that they don't fade out with stress and are consistent for at least a week.

- A judgement will also be needed on the personal relevancy of the responses. For example, minor left/right discrimination changes may not be so relevant in a person who has a severe pain related incapacity whereas they may be more relevant in a person with a much more minor problem. This is a clinical reasoning judgement.

These proposed 'normal' responses are also summarised in Figure 3.14A-E.

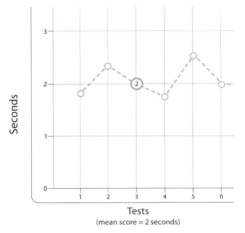

Figure 3.14A
The distribution of normal response times for left/right discrimination of the hands and feet.

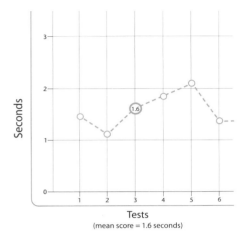

Figure 3.14B
The distribution of normal response times for left/right discrimination for backs and necks.

NOTE: *These normal distributions are based on studies of hundreds of people and act as a guide only. There may be reasons why, after months of practise, you still find it impossible to get results within these normal ranges. Aim for the normal range and give it a real go but don't be upset if you can't get there!*

GMI
hand
book

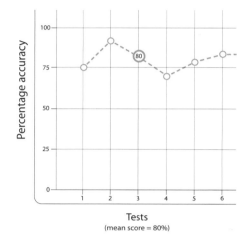

Figure 3.14C

The distribution of normal accuracy rate in left/right discrimination for hands.

(mean score = 85%)

3.14D

The distribution of normal accuracy rate in left/right discrimination for feet.

(mean score = 80%)

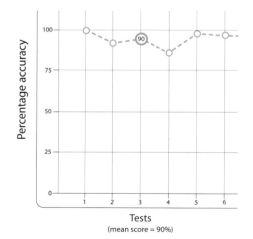

Figure 3.14E

The distribution of normal accuracy rate in left/right discrimination for neck and back.

(mean score = 90%)

4.3.4 Left/right discrimination for back and neck

Although we have mainly been discussing the limbs, left/right discrimination can also be performed for the back and the neck. The only difference is that you are guessing if the body part is moving (twisting, bending) to the left or to the right. Note in the discussion above on normal responses for the spine that the response times are usually faster than for the hands and feet. Rather than ask *'is this a left or right side of the neck?'*, the question to ask when viewing spine images such as Figure 3.12 is *'is this person turning his/her neck to the left or the right?'*

4.4. PATIENTS' AND THERAPISTS' STORIES ABOUT LEFT/RIGHT DISCRIMINATION EXERCISES

4.4.1 Guidance in progression in left/right judgement tasks

The GMI programme is still new and we find ourselves advising health practitioners as much as we do patients. We are all learning together. Rebecca is a physiotherapist looking for advice about how to use Recognise with her patients and in particular, how to progress with the programme as part of a treatment.

Rebecca: 'I can get my patients started, usually with about 20 images for 10 seconds. I select less images and longer times for the more sensitive patients, but I don't feel comfortable with when to move onto the following treatment and I always wonder if I am moving too fast or too slow. What guidelines can you give me for progressing my patients with left/right discrimination training?'

Tim: 'There is a bit of trial and error here and there are no hard and fast rules. Generally you can increase the number of pictures and reduce the amount of viewing time per picture, although not at the same time. When the accuracy and response time results are similar left to right, and fairly stable then change to context or abstract images. This is considered to be a progression in itself but isn't always. If you have changed the context of the image (making it harder) then it may be necessary to go back and show fewer images for slightly longer. This means that as you increase the difficulty of the image shown you keep the task manageable by reducing the difficulty elsewhere.

It is important for all users to have some basic understanding of how to progress with the programme. I recommend that you avoid changing too many parameters at once so that you allow the brain to get used to the changes. Rebecca is quite comfortable starting left/right discrimination testing and while she often starts with 20 vanilla images for 10 seconds, she will adapt this based on her initial assessment of the patient's sensitivity.

4.4.2 'Why is my right hand slower than the left?'

Rebecca still requires some guidance regarding the use of Recognise with her patient Linda, who has had persistent right wrist and arm pain for several years.

Rebecca: 'I have a few questions regarding the results on Recognise. Linda is working with 20 images for 5 seconds each. She is slightly more accurate with the right than the left although her response time is slower (accuracy is around 95% on the right and 92% on the left; speed is 2.0 seconds on the right and 1.3 on the left) Why is this so as it is her right arm that is the problem?'

Tim: 'It is likely that she is slower on the affected side due to a change in the representation of her right hand in the brain. During the test you mentally rotate the body part into that position and then confirm the choice. In people with hand pain it has been shown that they are accurate at working out the left from the right but are generally slower on the affected side. It could be that the change in representation of Linda's hand in her brain means it takes longer to mentally rotate the limb to mimic the picture and make the decision.

At the moment we don't know confidently why it is that with chronic hand and arm pain sufferers are more likely to present with slowing of their response times as opposed to a change in the accuracy. Lorimer makes some suggestions in his chapter, see chapter 2, Figure 2.3A-D.

4.4.3 Changing context and brain enrichment

Kate has had persistent right wrist and hand pain following a decompression operation for carpal tunnel syndrome two months earlier. She has spent a few weeks practicing her left/right discrimination for hands on Recognise and is beginning to see improvements in her results. She is also experiencing a reduction in her wrist and hand pain.

> **Kate:** 'On using Recognise, my speed has increased, as has my accuracy. Looking at my results the accuracy of right and left are coming closer together but I wonder how close do they need to be and what percentage of accuracy is acceptable before moving on? I am practicing with 30 pictures for 5 seconds, four sessions a day. How and when should I progress?'

> **Tim:** 'As long as the accuracy is 90% or above, the response times are below 2 seconds and the left/right accuracy and response times are reasonably similar then you are ready to move on. In terms of the left/right discrimination progression, you can either reduce the time that the images are viewed or increase the difficulty of the task in another way, such as changing the environment that you are practicing in. Why not try using Recognise at work too? Make sure you are also using the flash cards and magazines as well.'

Kate is progressing well and is beginning to see some positive results. One way of giving the flexibility and freedom back to the brain is to begin to change other elements of the test such as the environment or social situation (See Table 3.1). This will cause different areas of the brain to be activated, essentially exercising the pain neurotag in a good way.

- Length of display time for images
- Number of images
- Context of images – vanilla, context, abstract
- Where left/right judgements are performed – home, work, café.
- External environment – music or TV on in background, friend/therapist nearby
- Time of day (your brain chemistry changes throughout the day)
- Your mood (your brain will be enriched if you do the exercise in different moods)
- Different postures (try it on the floor or standing up)
- Do it in the nude if you want!

Table 3.1 *Possible environmental and contextual ideas for Recognise*

Jane has been also been looking for ways to increase the difficulty of the Recognise exercises. She has been experimenting with ways of altering the context of the exercise and therefore making the task either more or less difficult/threatening. This ties into her understanding of graded exposure.

> **Jane:** *'I turned the radio on and left it on as I would have done last year. This is normal for me, and I discovered it made the left/right discrimination test more difficult. I was pleased that I had taken a step forward, but am beginning to wonder if I over stimulated myself. I felt like I attended a day of complicated lectures and I felt brain drained. It may be a useful tool, but maybe I need a more measured approach?'*

> **Tim:** *'Having the radio on is a good example of how you can change the context of your brain training. Why not use it for just one of the sets of images e.g. the vanilla ones for now. Try building up to using it more so that you work towards increasing the amount of effort required as you go. Another way of building it up would be to start with music that you are familiar with and that you used to play and listen to before you had a problem. As a progression you could play music that you are not so familiar with or even dislike.'*

This shows just how hard the brain may need to work in order to process the images. It is important to realise that doing too much of this could cause a flare-up, particularly in people who are extremely sensitised. Jane's story also reminds us that brain exercise is hard work.

4.4.4 Incentivising left/right discrimination

Another great advantage of using the Recognise programme as part of training is the immediate feedback that it gives both the patient and clinician. The task really needs to be repeated often throughout the day (at least 4 or 5 times). For many patients (and clinicians) this can create a positive boost. Check out Tom's chapter to see how you can view the feedback from the results. Jane has really noticed a change in her pain and is enjoying using Recognise to exercise her left/right discrimination.

> **Jane:** *'Computer tests are brilliant, it's exciting to see how many consecutive results of 100% I can achieve and it's also a big motivator to see how I go after each test. This spurs me on when I'm getting tired!'*

As a clinician it can be really beneficial being able to look at your patients' results and where necessary to guide them. See Tom's chapter for information on how clinicians can view their patients' scores. Likewise for patients it can be a great incentive to know that someone is interested in how you are doing! In fact knowing that someone is monitoring your home exercise programme will increase the adherence to the programme[7].

4.4.5 Unusual responses

Sometimes you find unexpected test results. The first thing is not to panic and to maintain a flexible approach. Although we don't have the solid science to explain all the changes we find, some changes make sense from what we do know.

Kate: '*I'm viewing context hands, 30 images, 5 seconds, 5 or 6 sessions a day. I can't wait to see what I'll find next! I'm finding it much easier than vanilla hands, although the backgrounds and state of some of the hands in context hands are far more distracting. Why is this?'*

Tim: '*That is interesting. It may be that your brain finds it can relate to specific tasks and goals more easily to hands than when there is nothing to put them into context. This could be your mirror neurone system working, trying to understand essentially what the hand in the picture is doing.'*

It is interesting here that Kate finds context images easier than the vanilla ones. This may fit in with the results explained in the mirror neurone literature where there is increased activity of the mirror neurone system (discussed in Lorimer's chapter) during observation of goal and socially orientated tasks. We can learn from unusual responses – see David's section on 'out of the shadows learning' in chapter 1.

4.5 SUMMARY OF LEFT/RIGHT DISCRIMINATION TASKS

Left/right discrimination tasks are a great way to assess changes in the unconscious representation of body movements and body parts. The Recognise programme provides one avenue for assessing these changes but magazines and flash cards can also be used as alternative tools. Changes to either response time and/or accuracy of the task can be identified in many different pain states like CRPS, phantom limb pain, back pain, neck pain and chronic leg and arm pain.

If there is a problem identified using left/right discrimination then it is possible to use the same methods to improve it. These exercises need to be performed in an unconscious manner, so that it will feel more like you're guessing as you will be working so quickly. By maintaining this approach it is hoped that you will exercise the brain without activating the pain neurotag.

Let's now look at stage 2 of the graded motor imagery progression - explicit motor imagery.

5. EXPLICIT MOTOR IMAGERY

5.1 INTRODUCTION AND DEFINITION

Motor imagery is an imagined movement or in the language of neuroscience – the self-generated representation (neurotag) in your brain of a movement or posture without actually performing the movement or posture. It is a process in which you are aware of yourself thinking about what you are doing, therefore we call it 'explicit'.

We can all imagine performing a movement and putting our bodies in certain postures. Before a golfer putts, he or she will imagine the action and the ball going into the hole. Mountain climbers imagine themselves at the top of the mountain. There is good evidence that imagining an athletic performance first will improve the actual performance. Surgeons who imagine a surgical procedure first will have better mastery over their surgical performance[3].

This section focuses on motor imagery, or imagining movements and postures. However, imagery can also involve taste (imagining a taste), hearing (imagining a sound), smell and touch. Utilisation of these sensations may well have a place in the brain retraining that we suggest in GMI or may enhance the process of motor imagery.

5.1.1 The power of imagery

Imagining movements can be hard work. Your heart rate can change just through imagining movements. Your capacity to perform explicit motor imagery is dependent on you as an individual and your environment (both real and imagined), just as actually moving would be[13]. The time taken to perform the same actual and imagined tasks would be roughly the same.

Consider walking along a path or imagining walking along the same path – it should take the same amount of time. If you then had to walk along a narrow line on this path, such as a balance beam, this takes longer both actually walking along it and imagining walking along it. Your brain therefore adjusts to the task.

Just as a change in the task or environment alters our ability to perform imagined movements so does the position you are in when you do it. The same task of imagining walking along a path would be more difficult to do if you do the imagining whilst you are holding your leg bent up as opposed to standing straight. There are obvious clinical implications for the user to draw from these examples when deciding to perform motor imagery.

5.2 OBSERVING, IMAGINING AND PERFORMING MOVEMENT

There is a small difference in the extent of activation of the motor areas such that observing movement broadly activates these areas less than imagining moving and in turn, imagining moving activates them less than performing the actual movement (Figure 3.15).

As Figure 3.15 implies, onset of the pain neurotag in someone who experiences pain during left/right discrimination activities might be avoided by using simple observation of the movement. Lorimer discusses the possible science behind this in his chapter.

5.3 THE TOOLS FOR EXPLICIT MOTOR IMAGERY

Motor imagery is not only powerful, it is free and you can do it anywhere. In fact it is a good thing for the brain to do it in as many different places as possible. The main tools you need are knowledge, some basic techniques and some notions of progression. These are all illustrated below in patients' stories.

Recognise is also designed for explicit motor imagery. You can set up your own motor imagery tests and adjust viewing time, kind of image and insert your own images. Tom takes you through this in chapter 5.

Flash cards can be used in much the same way as Recognise as they provide movements or postures to imagine. These could fit well with a structured graded exposure approach, particularly if you have identified a fear hierarchy as discussed earlier in this chapter (Figure 3.9). Recall that we discussed earlier how the rotation of the image would impact on the speed and accuracy of the test.

Magazines or photographs are some of the other tools that can be used. They may help you to imagine moving like someone else or to remember how you moved previously (although this may require some care). There are obviously many different tools that can be used as adjuncts and some of these will be discussed below. Hopefully though, the reader will recognise that just sitting in a mall watching people walking by is a form of explicit motor imagery.

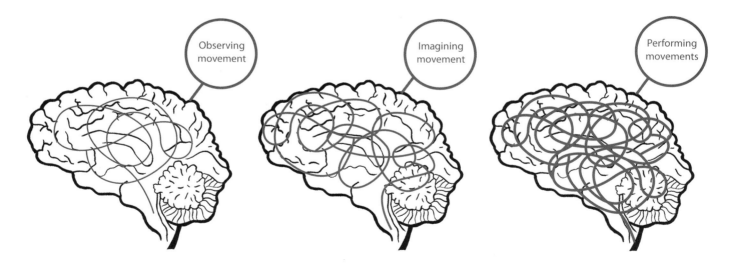

Figure 3.15 *The increased degree of activation of motor and other areas in the brain when observing, imagining and performing movement.*

5.4 THE PROCESS ILLUSTRATED VIA PATIENT STORIES

Starting the explicit motor imagery process takes preparation just as it would to start any exercise. This includes a little direction in terms of instructions for how to perform motor imagery. As a general rule, explicit motor imagery is a first person exercise, which means you are imagining yourself in a particular posture or doing the movement. It is also supposed to be more of a sense of 'feeling' that you are doing it, rather than 'seeing' it. Try this:

> 'Think about your right shoulder and where it is in space. Really put all your thoughts into your right shoulder. Perhaps you can feel a bit of clothing touching it or some air blowing over it. Maybe you can sense the way your arm hangs down from your shoulder.'

Most people are able to take themselves through this and experience a heightened awareness of their right shoulder in the particular posture that they find themselves. Let's now consider the shoulder moving:

> 'Bring your thoughts back to your right shoulder. Close your eyes now and imagine reaching forward to pick up a glass. Do this slowly and as you do this keep your thoughts on how your shoulder feels. Perhaps you are aware of it moving as a part of the whole movement of your arm or you can sense the movement just from your shoulder.'

You may have to repeat this or try it on other body parts that you find easier to imagine. Most people will be able to sense how it feels to move or at least how a body part feels in a particular position. There are exceptions, especially if you are in pain, so there are ways to maximise the effect when you are struggling to perform motor imagery in this way.

5.4.1 'Get me started!'

Jane, who has CRPS1 of her left foot, is ready to begin motor imagery.

> **Jane:** 'Could you explain how to visualise a limb and which limb I should start with and for how long I need to do it?'
>
> **Tim:** 'I would begin with the unaffected leg. Imagine your leg and the position it is in. Feel the air around it or how your sock presses gently into it. Take your thoughts up and down your leg.
>
> You may be best to begin this process higher up the leg before progressing down towards the toes. At the moment I wouldn't imagine doing any movement with the affected leg or you could even try going through this process on your hand first to see how it feels.'

It is a good idea to try motor imagery on a body part away from the affected area (so not the painful spot). This will enable the user to experience some mastery of the task and subsequent feedback on how it should feel. Work towards the affected area by starting away from it to begin with.

5.4.2 'I just can't visualise!'

Kate who has right wrist and hand pain following surgery for carpal tunnel syndrome has been practising left/right discrimination on Recognise for several weeks. She is seeing an improvement in terms of the level of her pain and also her sleep. However, she is struggling to visualise her affected arm and hand.

> **Kate:** *'I have started on the motor imagery but cannot visualise my right hand and arm. It's as if I know that the (right) hand on the table must be mine, but I can't see it. I can see my left hand and arm on the table but not the right hand and arm. What does this mean and what is the way forward?'*

> **Tim:** *'It is likely to tie in to the change in the representation of your hand and arm in your brain. To make this task easier I would begin by imagining your left arm first and spend a short time on the right. Another way would be to work down the right arm from areas that you can imagine. For now, try to get a sense of how it feels to do this.'*

Moseley[9] has demonstrated a similar finding in people with back pain. When they were asked to draw where they imagined their backs to be they often missed out or misrepresented the symptomatic area. When asked why, they reported that they had *'lost their back'* or *'couldn't find it'*. His theory to reason for this was an alteration of their body image brought about by their ongoing pain state.

5.4.3 'My body or someone else's?'

John, who has persistent neck pain, has tried many forms of traditional and alternative therapies, all of which have either given temporary relief or made his pain worse. His results on Recognise for left/right discrimination of the neck are very good so he is now beginning to go through explicit motor imagery exercises. He is very sensitive and visualising himself in the first person is just too difficult at the moment. Therefore, he is beginning to try motor imagery in the third person, in other words imagining someone else moving.

> **John:** *'For imagery, I am trying to concentrate on the flash card images without relating them directly to myself. I find this quite difficult but I am persevering. I can still feel a slight reaction but this is lessening. Is this the best way to go at the moment?'*

> **Tim:** *'You could persevere, but you could also try watching someone move and concentrate on their head and neck. This should be more comfortable and less threatening.'*

It is a good idea to use flash cards to establish a fear hierarchy as previously mentioned to find out if there are certain positions that are more or less threatening. It may be appropriate to take a further step back and one way to do this would be to watch someone else move. This will still activate brain areas involved in movement but to a lesser extent than going through imagined movements yourself, so that the pain neurotag will not be activated or further sensitised whilst promoting some inhibition (dampening down) of the sensitised brain areas.

5.4.4 Taking a step back

There are times when someone becomes so sensitised that it takes some effort and significant collaboration between the patient and the clinician to work out a suitable baseline to start activity.

Claire has back and leg pain that affects all of her movements. She needs to take a step back in her treatment process. Look at her comment and see how it leads us towards an approach that is more targeted to the brain.

> *Claire: 'I definitely need some ideas to make me feel happier thinking about moving. Watching a video of me walking is too scary to even think about.'*

Claire is a great example of someone whose pain neurotag has become highly sensitised. Just thinking about moving or even watching herself move is sufficient to activate fear associated with moving. It is important to recognise this and as a reasoner, find ways to step back a little.

> *Tim: 'Why not actively watch people moving for short periods until you feel happy with that for now. You can adjust the distance that you are away from them too. The closer you are, the more sensitive you may be.'*

It is likely that just watching people move will give the brain some enrichment and be not as much work for the brain as imagining movements.

5.4.5 'Can I hurt myself with imagery?'

Claire has gone through a process of observing other people move and is happy with the thought of herself moving now. She has started imagined movements from a first person perspective but her pain neurotag is still highly sensitive and easily ignited.

> *Claire: 'I have been doing imagined movements for about five minutes at a time during different times of the day. Is there any benefit to be gained from stirring things up now or is it best to stop very quickly when this happens?'*
>
> *Tim: 'It is OK to be a bit sore as long as you're not flaring yourself up. Try to work within your baseline limit that you have set yourself. As you change your exercises your brain needs to get used to the new challenges so it is usual for someone to feel a bit sensitive to begin with. This will settle as your brain feels happier and more accustomed to the exercises.'*

When someone has a sensitised pain neurotag it is important to retain your knowledge of the graded exposure approach. Here is where the twin peaks model (discussed by David in chapter 4 of this book) can be used and in particular, use of the mantra that 'it is OK to be sore as long as you are safe'. This is a mantra that often needs to be reinforced. The pain sufferer (or the clinician) would have a goal in mind to practise these mantras within the buffer zone. An example may be to practice some explicit motor imagery tasks and aim to stay under a pain score of 2 out of 10 during this activity. If this was achieved for a week without any blips or increases in pain scores it could be used as a guide for moving forward to more threatening cards, movements or contexts.

5.4.6 Context change and graded exposure in explicit motor imagery

I recommend finding ways to strengthen the process of explicit motor imagery by changing cues and descriptions. This essential part of the motor imagery process is called contextualisation. Not only does it help to enhance the process but it also fits into the graded exposure process aimed at giving freedom and flexibility back to the brain.

Kate is experimenting with changes in context during her imagined movements.

> *Kate:* '*I wondered could I take one element such as thinking about the air around my hand to help the imagery process?*'

> *Tim:* '*Yes I think this is a good idea. It requires experimenting, finding what is most comforting and aids the imagery process. There are many different ways of helping the imagery process and enhancing the feeling of your body in a positive way.*'

Jane had exceptional left/right discrimination scores but when she moved onto explicit motor imagery concentrating on the affected leg was too much. As a result she began imagining movements which did not involve the affected area. She occasionally included her affected leg in the motor imagery but tried not to focus on it.

> *Jane:* '*I wondered if I should imagine my hand in situations that are more stimulating to my leg e.g. wheeling my wheelchair outside in the dark? That way my hand passes by my leg during the imagery.*'

> *Tim:* '*That sounds to be a great way of including your leg in the imagery process. Let me know any further thoughts so we can understand better what to do and how to include your leg in the imagery process.*'

Changes in the context in which the task is performed will affect the response to that task. Following the principles of graded exposure, the aim would be to begin with altering small aspects of the explicit motor imagery process in order to find the least threatening or pain provoking method. This will avoid over stimulating the pain neurotag and maintaining sensitisation. The user can progress through imagery to challenge the brain as sensitisation reduces. Examples of ways to alter the context of motor imagery exercises are presented in Table 3.2.

- Where do I practice explicit motor imagery? At home, work, school, on the bus, in the bath?

- Do I keep my eyes open or closed during motor imagery?

- What position do I adopt during imagery? Sitting, standing, lying?

- Do I think of myself moving (first person) or someone else moving (third person)?

- How long should I perform imagery for and how many times a day?

- What is the task complexity and intensity and how does it tie in with grading my exposure?

- What words should the therapist use to describe or talk through the process?

- What words should the user think of when going through the process?

- Should there be prior demonstration of the movement by another person (therapist, family member)?

- What cues can be used to heighten the process? Sounds, memories, smells?

- Do I use relaxation or meditation in conjunction?

- How much do I know about the changes in the brain that I can achieve with imagery?

Table 3.2 Some questions the user could be asking him or herself and ideas for contextualising explicit motor imagery

These are questions for which there are no wrong or right answers but that give you some ideas to work from.

There are endless variations that can be incorporated into the explicit motor imagery process. This allows creativity for the user and aims to give freedom and flexibility back to the brain.

5.5   SUMMARY OF EXPLICIT MOTOR IMAGERY

Explicit motor imagery is essentially thinking about moving without actually moving. There are many different ways to go through the process and the most common method used in GMI is a first person perspective of feeling your own movement.

Explicit motor imagery fits well into the graded exposure approach of GMI as a result of the altered activation of the motor areas in the brain. Broadly speaking there is greater activation during explicit motor imagery than implicit motor imagery (left/right discrimination). Observation of movement may provide another way of stepping back when the pain neurotag is highly sensitised.

Contextual change is important in all forms of rehabilitation and training. The choices required to reason through the use of explicit motor imagery highlight the creativity possible within GMI and link well with the aim of giving the brain back what it wants – flexibility and freedom.

We're now going to explore the use of mirrors as stage 3 of the graded motor imagery programme.

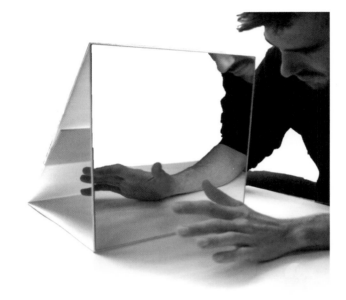

6.   MIRRORS – 'THE USER AS ILLUSIONIST'

6.1   INTRODUCTION AND DEFINITION

Mirrors, as with imagery have been used in rehabilitation for many years but it was more recently that Ramachandran and Rogers-Ramachandran explored their use for phantom limb pain[12]. Their initial research showed that there were clear signs that using mirrors could benefit complex pain states and that the target was likely to be the brain. As Lorimer said, this is really what stimulated his research into GMI.

Essentially mirror therapy means looking into a mirror to see the reflection of the limb held in front of it (Figure 3.16). The mirror will effectively give the illusion that you are looking at the limb that is hidden.

The brain activation during the use of mirrors is less than actual movement but slightly more compared with imagining the same movement. This ties into the graded exposure approach that GMI follows.

Interestingly the people who experience the greatest pain relief following mirror therapy are those who have an ability to imagine moving their affected limb[14]. This emphasises the need to have intact motor imagery ability in order to gain the greatest benefit.

Figure 3.16 Using a mirror box. In this situation the problematic right hand is hidden in the box. Looking at the mirror image of the left hand gives the illusion of seeing the hidden right hand.

6.2 THE TOOLS FOR MIRROR THERAPY

For mirror therapy the most important piece of equipment is a good mirror. This means one that gives a true reflection of the body part so that it doesn't look like you've stepped into the house of mirrors in the circus. There is compelling evidence that if someone sees the reflection of a larger or wibbly-wobbly limb it may make his or her pain worse[11].

You can make your own mirror box or there are commercial mirror boxes available. On safety grounds, we recommend using a good quality perspex mirrors rather than glass. The NOI Mirror Box is great for hand and wrist problems due to its good quality mirror, collapsibility and portability. This means that the user can transport it easily and use it in different contexts such as at work or in the café. It may be important to use a longer mirror for feet, legs and arms, so that there is less need to bend over to see the reflection. A longer mirror also provides a fuller reflection of a leg. It is more difficult to use a mirror for the treatment of neck and back problems for obvious reasons (Figure 3.18A-D).

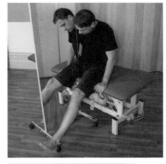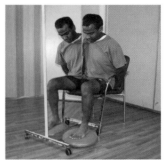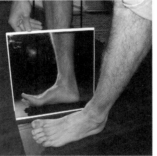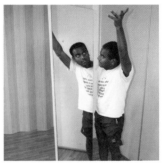

| *Figure 3.18A-D* *Examples of mirrors used in clinics.*

Treatment through Graded Motor Imagery
www.noigroup.com

GMI
hand
book

6.3   STARTING THE PROCESS

For some people this illusion is so real that it can be quite a shock to begin with. The clinician should appropriately prepare patients before having them try. In the same way that left/right discrimination and explicit motor imagery can be started in a different part of the body to the affected area so can using mirrors. The clinician could begin by demonstrating what is involved. Make the environment as de-threatening as possible. You may not want a pack of students watching a patient with severe pain, trying out mirror therapy for the first time!

To get the most out of the illusion it is important to make it believable. This may mean taking off jewellery, watches or covering tattoos. There is an obvious problem here for the bilateral amputee (although this may be solved with the use of a prosthetic limb).

For most body parts, it is best started in a seated position with the mirror placed roughly in the midline of the body and so that the user can look into the mirror and see a reflection of the body part in front of it (Figure 3.16). The process involves accommodating and accepting the reflection and allowing the brain to be lured into the illusion. This may take seconds or may require some prompting, just like the cues that can be used to enhance the explicit motor imagery process.

As with each part of the GMI process it is important to consider the sensitivity of the pain neurotag. It may be appropriate to start with a very safe exercise despite previously working at a challenging level with explicit or conscious motor imagery. To begin with, this may mean keeping the limb still both inside and outside of the mirror box. Moving the limb outside of the mirror box whilst keeping the hidden one static is a logical progression. A further progression would be moving the hidden limb within its baseline limit whilst taking the other limb through large movements. A final progression would be to move both limbs equally (see Table 3.3 for a summary and more suggestions).

In general we consider it appropriate to keep the movements congruous or the same once the hand in the box is able to move. This means that your brain isn't getting too many mixed messages. It may be that the mixed messages are sufficient to set off a pain neurotag[5].

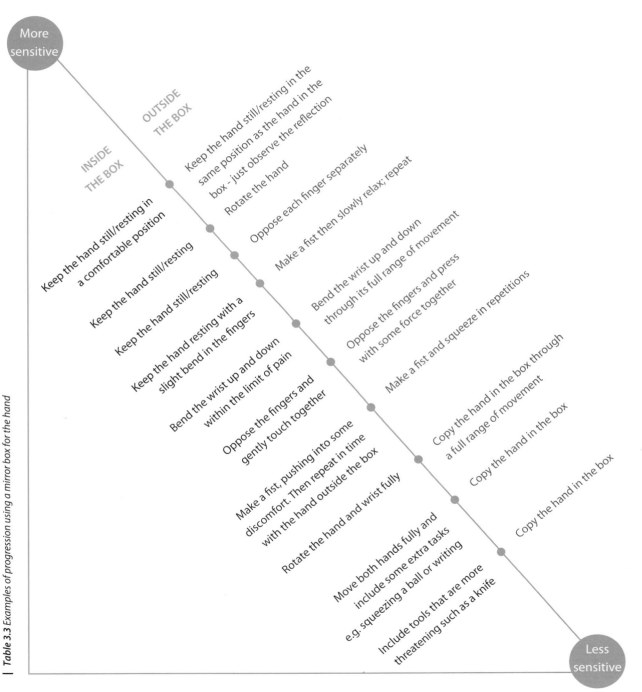

| *Table 3.3 Examples of progression using a mirror box for the hand*

More sensitive

Less sensitive

INSIDE THE BOX

OUTSIDE THE BOX

Keep the hand still/resting in a comfortable position

Keep the hand still/resting in the same position as the hand in the box - just observe the reflection

Keep the hand still/resting

Rotate the hand

Keep the hand still/resting with a slight bend in the fingers

Oppose each finger separately

Make a fist then slowly relax; repeat

Bend the wrist up and down within the limit of pain

Bend the wrist up and down through its full range of movement

Oppose the fingers and gently touch together

Oppose the fingers and press with some force together

Make a fist, pushing into some discomfort. Then repeat in time with the hand outside the box

Make a fist and squeeze in repetitions

Rotate the hand and wrist fully

Copy the hand in the box through a full range of movement

Copy the hand in the box

Move both hands fully and include some extra tasks e.g. squeezing a ball or writing

Copy the hand in the box

Include tools that are more threatening such as a knife

GMI
hand
book

6.4   THE PROCESS – PATIENT STORIES

The use of mirrors in rehabilitation is often easier to market than the previous components of the Graded Motor Imagery process. The mirror is an actual device, whereas the left/right judgements and motor imagery can be a bit abstract. Mirrors are familiar and you will be sure to get at least some response when you use the box.

6.4.1 Starting in a static position and the use of Flash cards

Rebecca has been working through the GMI process with her patient Linda. Linda has experienced right hand and wrist pain for several years. Operations on both her wrist and elbow gave little relief. She has worked through the process of implicit and explicit motor imagery and found a reduction in pain and improvement in her function. Now she has moved on to using mirrors.

> **Rebecca:** 'Linda can only tolerate 1-2 minutes of keeping her right hand in the mirror box while moving her left hand. I have told her to stop moving the left and just keep it in the different static positions that bother the right. While doing this she is keeping the right still in its most comfortable position so that the brain gets used to seeing her 'right hand 'in these positions. How would you progress from here?'

> **Tim:** 'This sounds like good advice. I would suggest you start with easier static positions to hold the left hand in first. You can gradually progress to the harder or more threatening ones as Linda gets used to it – perhaps you could use a fear hierarchy to direct you with the progression. Keep it at 1-2 minutes for now as you let her brain get used to the more comfortable positions. Check the environment of the mirror exercises as well – it should be done in a peaceful place at this stage'.

It was a good idea to stop moving the hand when looking at the reflections and just get used to static positions. However, if Linda's pain neurotag was highly sensitive it may not have been necessary or advisable to work into the bothersome positions. Using flash cards as a way of planning your progression through movements and exercises in the mirror creates some structure.

6.4.2 Remember to work within baselines and avoid flare-ups

Claire has worked through GMI following a leg injury and although highly sensitive has been working to a challenging degree with her explicit motor imagery. She has been using left/right discrimination as a settling exercise throughout the day but is getting a little bored with the exercises and is keen to move on to using mirrors.

> **Claire:** 'I had a strong reaction on Friday from using the mirror for too long. Actually it didn't surprise me, I knew I was pushing it. I have backed off and have tried the mirror for very short periods. I can now see my foot very quickly and accept it.'

> **Tim:** 'It is important that you don't move past your baseline and flare your pain up. You've done the right

thing by reducing the amount of time. Also remind yourself that although you have had some pain, it is extremely unlikely that you will have caused any damage.'

Even though you may have moved forward in terms of the GMI sequence, you still need to remember the initial principles of baselines, patience and persistence.

6.4.3 Context can alter mirror responses

Claire is experimenting with contextualisation in order to find the most comfortable use of mirrors.

> **Claire:** *'I feel I can use the mirror longer when I have music playing in the background.'*

> **Tim:** *'Great! It sounds like you've found a way of playing a different neurotag. Make sure you try it with all kinds of music, not just your favourite music.'*

Graded exposure works well with contextualisation. Seemingly small changes in the environment can have profound effects. This is great for the more sensitised pain states.

Different music can affect our moods and therefore our physiology. Perhaps you would start with calmer, happier music and then work towards more stimulating music in order to challenge your ability during a stressful situation. Remember the different contextual changes that have been mentioned previously. For example mirror therapy could be carried out at different times of the day, you could use tools (pens, cutlery, kicking a ball for the foot), do it in different states of mind. There are many ways to perform the same activity in the mirror, it just requires creativity.

6.4.4 Instant relief in a mirror?

Pam is in her 60s and has recently had her plaster cast removed from her left wrist. She has fractured it in a fall 6 weeks previously. She has had constant pain that is aggravated by all movements of her hand and wrist. She has also had visible swelling and changes in the appearance of her skin. Dark hair growth has appeared over the back of the wrist.

Pam was prescribed general range of movement exercises one week ago, but was unable to do these due to the pain. She tried performing the same movements but this time with the injured hand behind the mirror. As soon as she saw the reflection of her right hand in the mirror she experienced temporary relief of the pain in her left hand and wrist. Following several attempts she was able to move the right and left hand in synchrony with greater ease whilst using the mirror.

Pain relief was maintained with daily practice over the next four weeks. All other changes such as swelling, skin appearance and hair growth improved steadily over this time. She recovered hand function and was able to go back to her work at a jewellery shop.

There are times, particularly with more acute pain problems that mirrors by themselves have been used beneficially[6]. For the user it requires some reasoning in order to appropriately choose when to either move on with each part of the GMI process or whether to skip any.

6.5   SUMMARY – USING MIRRORS

Mirrors can be an effective and powerful tool. They have been used independently to help reduce pain and improve movement and function. It is the ability to create an illusion that is so powerful and allows the activation of the movement areas of the brain in a graded way, thus avoiding awakening the pain neurotag. Broadly speaking there is a slight increase in this activation in comparison with explicit motor imagery. This suggests it is appropriate to follow motor imagery as part of the GMI programme.

Contextual change can be used in the same way as left/right discrimination and explicit motor imagery. Contextualisation allows a continuation of graded exposure. As with the two previous elements there is potential for it to be used in a variety of settings and this adds flexibility, something that the brain loves!

Let's see now how these fit together as a sequential process.

7.   GRADED MOTOR IMAGERY AS A WHOLE – DON'T BE SATISFIED WITH JUST MANAGING PAIN

The overriding principle of the GMI process is that it is a treatment aimed at giving flexibility and creativity back to the brain in order to promote health and wellbeing. It appears necessary that this treatment be provided in a sequential manner. In other words someone must have intact implicit motor imagery (or be able to easily and rapidly judge left from right), prior to moving onto the explicit stage of motor imagery, which in turn they must train before beginning with mirror therapy[8]. There are many studies that look at the provision of one component of the GMI process and treatment by itself but limited research looking at the whole process.

As suggested with Pam following her wrist fracture, it may be appropriate to skip stages of the process. However, this requires further investigation, as it is impossible to know that she wouldn't have benefited more from going through left/right discrimination and/or explicit motor imagery. The instant relief and subsequent rapid recovery however, suggests it was an appropriate strategy with such an acute case.

It appears with recent evidence that intact left/right discrimination is lost in many different pain states (see chapter 2). As such, it may be necessary to re-establish it, or at the very least assess for any disturbance in it before moving forwards with treatment and rehabilitation.

A fear hierarchy essentially means finding out the order from the least to the most feared activity. This may mean changing the context of the activity (such as your mood state or the environment). It could also mean finding out specific movements that are expected to be more or less difficult (or painful). This can help guide the graded part of the process. You can be creative when working out the changes in context. Just consider how the activity fits into interests, home life, environment or alternatively what sets off the pain neurotag.

It's exciting to think that in the future, the development of many chronic pain problems may be avoided, and sufferers may be offered effective treatment. Time to get your brains fizzing!

GMI
hand
book

REFERENCES

1. Bowering J, Butler DS, Fulton I, et al. Implicit motor imagery in people with a history of back pain, current back pain, both or neither. Submitted 2012.

2. Butler DS, Moseley GL. *Explain Pain*. Adelaide: Noigroup Publications, 2003.

3. DesCoteaux JG, Leclere H. Learning surgical technical skills. Canadian Journal of Surgery 1995;38:33-8.

4. Leeuw M, Goossens MEJB, sde Jong J, et al. The fear-avoidance model of musculoskeletal pain: Current state of scientific evidence. Journal of Behavioral Medicine 2007;30:77-94.

5. McCabe CS, Haigh RC, Halligan PW, et al. Simulating sensory-motor incongruence in healthy volunteers: implications for a cortical model of pain Rheumatology 2005;44:509-16.

6. McCabe CS, Haigh RC, Ring EFR, et al. A controlled pilot study of the utility of mirror visual feedback in the treatment of complex regional pain syndrome (type 1). Rheumatology (Oxford) 2003;42:97-101.

7. Moseley GL. Do training diaries affect and reflect adherence to home programs? Arthritis and Rheumatism 2006;55:662-4.

8. Moseley GL. Graded motor imagery for pathologic pain. Neurology 2006;67:1-6.

9. Moseley GL. I can't find it! Distorted body image and tactile dysfunction in patients with chronic low back pain. Pain 2008;140:239-43.

10. Moseley GL. Is successful rehabilitation of complex regional pain syndrome due to sustained attention to the affected limb. Pain 2005;114:54-61.

11. Moseley GL, Parsons TJ, Spence T. Visual distortion of a limb modulats the pain and swelling evoked by movement Curent Biology 2009;18:R1047-8.

12. Ramachandran VS, Rogers- Ramachandran D. Synaesthesia in phantom limbs induced with mirrors. Proceedings of the Royal Society of London B. 1996;236:377-86.

13. Stevens JA. Interference effects demonstrate distinct roles for visual and motor imagery during the mental representation of human action. Cognition 2005;95:329-50.

14. Sumitani M, Miyauchi S, McCabe CS, et al. Mirror visual feedback alleviates deafferentation pain, dependimng on qualitative aspects of the pain: a preliminary report. Rheumatology 2008;47:1038-43.

15. Vlaeyen JWS, Linton SJ. Fear-avoidance and its consequences in chronic musculoskeletal pain: a state of the art. Pain 2000;85:317-22.

16. Wallwork S, Butler DS, Darmawan I, et al. Motor Imagery of the neck. Age, gender, handedness and image rotation affect performace on a left/right neck rotation judgement task. Submitted 2012.

NOTES

Helping the Graded Motor Imagery process with stories and metaphors

David S. Butler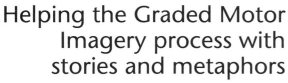

1. INTRODUCTION

In the first chapter I discussed the importance of gaining as much knowledge as possible about pain and the GMI process and how a good information base could be critical to your outcome. The last two chapters have provided an enormous amount of information about GMI research and its practical applications.

Let's now return to some more practical applications of learning.

2. METAPHORS AND STORIES

When you sit around a dinner table and someone tells the same story again and again, if you listen instead of yawning or walking out, you may notice that the story changes slightly each time. We all construct stories of the innumerable aspects of our lives and this includes our health and pain experiences as we give it a language which we tweak over time. While some may be a literal story, much of this story that we make will be in metaphors. We not only express ourselves in metaphors (*'that doctor has a heart of gold'; 'he is a pain in the arse'*), it's also how we learn and pick up information quickly, whether right or wrong (*'no pain no gain'*). There are different kinds of metaphors too. For example, the common metaphor equating one thing with another that we have been discussing (*'he is as strong as an ox'*) and ontological metaphors where we try to give meaning to abstract concepts such as the mind (*'he has very fragile mind'*) and pain (*'it hurts like hell, it hit me like a ton of bricks'*)[6].

These metaphors and the story they support can 'become us'. They will have their own neurotags in the brain and we produce them just like we produce pain, movements, sweats and emotions. Our stories give us meaning. They are us.

2.1 WHAT DOES IT HAVE TO DO WITH GMI?

For an effective GMI process, I believe that it's good to have a store of both helpful metaphors (e.g. *'use it or lose it'*), to be aware of unhelpful metaphors (e.g. *'ignorance is bliss'*, *'no pain no gain'*), to have metaphors to help us ponder and reflect on our pain (e.g. *'pain as a defender not an offender'*) and to keep us going when things get hard (e.g. *'when the going gets tough, the tough get going'*). I also think that useful metaphors can be powered up for better effect and deep learning. For example, take *'motion is lotion'*. If this was left as a statement then it will just be a glib saying or heuristic like you see in the superficial learning pathway discussed in chapter 1. However the metaphor can be enriched or 'powered up' as we like to say, by knowledge about the beneficial effects of motion on your tissues, removing swelling, pumping blood and nourishing the brain. I'll talk about this later.

Lorimer wrote a great little book called *Painful Yarns*[7]. It's all about key pieces of knowledge for understanding pain, all enclosed in great stories – kind of long metaphors. It's worth a read, because the material in it has been looked at scientifically[3] and it is known to help.

Here are some metaphors and sayings that may be appropriate for you.

3. PROBLEM SOLVING METAPHORS AND SAYINGS TO GET YOU THROUGH

3.1 HELPFUL METAPHORS

There are many useful metaphors and stories to help you with a chronic pain state. I have picked three of our most commonly used ones. No one knows where these metaphors have come from – some surely from patients, others from the many clinicians we have trained and some have been handed down over time. We would also like to hear about metaphors that you have found helpful.

3.1.1 Motion is lotion

'Motion is lotion' has already been mentioned. It has been with us for many years and many Australian Physiotherapists use it. But it needs 'powering up' or supplemented with some literal stories to strengthen it and to place it deeper in the brain. I may say something like… *'if you can do those few exercises and movements that we discussed, you will put a nice coating of oil on your joint surfaces, move some old fluid out of your muscles, give "instructions" to your tissues about how to heal, make your blood thinner and nourish and exercise brain cells to make them fire better'.*

The idea that thinking of movement is a lotion for areas of brain that have not moved appropriately for some time and that the lotion gets them ready for real movement may be useful for some GMI users.

You can obviously adapt it as you wish. Seeking more information behind sayings is one way in which you can 'deep learn'. *'Motion is lotion'* goes nicely with *'use it or lose it'* or *'your next position is your best position'*. *'Use it or lose it'* is the same for synapses as it is for muscle strength.

3.1.2 'If you keep stepping back you will hit the wall'

In persistent pain states and particularly ones where there have been no relief and no information offered, people often keep stepping back from everything that hurts. While this may be appropriate with an acute injury, it is not appropriate for the long term and certainly not for a GMI user, even though initially it is understandable. Note in Figure 4.1, how if you keep stepping back, you will eventually have very little activity reserve at all. Pain usually needs to be teased, challenging and coaxing away at its edges. It is almost inevitable if you are using parts of the GMI programme, that any pain experienced will be due to central sensitisation – a very real and measurable pain related more to changes in synapses in the central nervous system than processes at the endings of nerves. It does not signal danger to tissues. Central sensitisation is discussed later in this chapter and in the next metaphor.

3.1.3 'Although I am sore I am safe'

Many patients and clinicians report that the most helpful image and associated story in the book *Explain Pain*[1] is the 'twin peaks model'. We have reproduced it below in Figure 4.2. Lorimer and I drew this image in 2002 while we were having a few beers in Sydney, before the GMI strategies were researched. We used it for actual movement, but it is as helpful for the imagery strategies in GMI. I have used it below to illustrate the metaphor *'sore but safe'*.

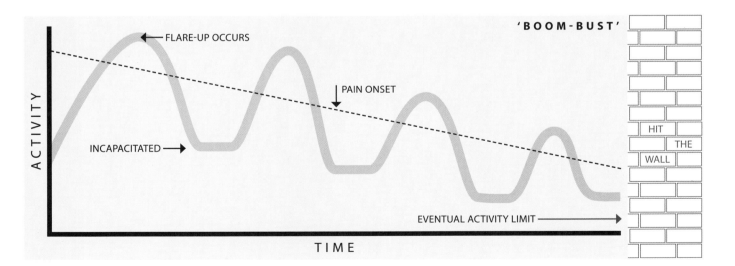

FLARE-UP OCCURS

'BOOM-BUST'

PAIN ONSET

ACTIVITY

INCAPACITATED

HIT THE WALL

EVENTUAL ACTIVITY LIMIT

TIME

Figure 4.1 If you keep stepping back you will eventually hit the wall. From Butler DS, Moseley, GL 2003 Explain Pain Noigroup Publications, Adelaide (with permission).

www.noigroup.com

Helping the Graded Motor Imagery process with stories and metaphors

GMI
hand
book

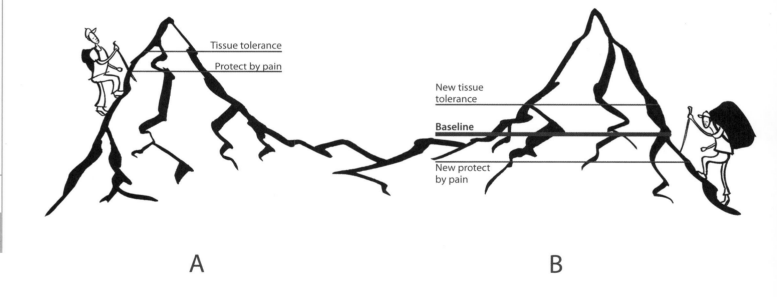

Tissue tolerance

Protect by pain

New tissue
tolerance

Baseline

New protect
by pain

A

B

Figure 4.2 *The twin peaks model with backpackers.*
Adapted from Butler DS, Moseley GL 2003 Explain Pain,
Noigroup Publications, Adelaide (with permission).

Figure A is the before pain state. You probably could have climbed a mountain before your problems started (or sat in a chair for 2 days to finish some writing, or walked for 10 kilometres). Let's imagine a mountain for now. If you keep climbing a mountain, you are likely to overuse, stretch and strain muscles and ligaments (note the 'tissue injury' line). But note also how the presence of pain is a warning – the 'protect by pain' line is below tissue injury so you will experience pain before the tissues are damaged. Note the backpacker and how there is not much in the backpack (injury, weakness, fears) holding them back.

Figure B could be where you are now. Note first that the 'tissue tolerance' is not quite as good as it was in A. While you have probably had plenty of time to heal (smashed bones can heal quite well in 6 weeks), your muscles, joints and other soft tissues are probably underused, sensitive and it's fair to say a 'bit out of condition' and 'in need of a good workout'.

Check how the 'protect by pain line' is quite low on the mountain compared to A. Basically your brain is doing a wonderful job of protecting you and it's now making pain when you climb a small mountain or maybe even when you think of climbing a mountain. The key issue is that the gap or buffer between the 'protect by pain line' and 'tissue injury line' is much wider in B. *Can you see how you could walk up part of the mountain, experience pain, or think about walking up the mountain, but that you are unlikely to hurt your tissues as you would need to go a long way in pain before you reach the place on the mountain where your tissues would be damaged.* Note that the backpack is bigger on the climber on Figure B, making it harder to climb. If you are a sufferer you may want to ask – what is in your backpack right now? Fitness, flexibility, knowledge, anger, lack of direction etc etc. Can you make your backpack a little lighter?

If you are a GMI user and have a sensitive pain state such as Complex Regional Pain Syndrome, you are unlikely to be climbing mountains or running marathons (yet). Your mountain may be a small movement or more likely, thinking of a movement. It may help to think that the difference between thinking of a movement and actually performing a movement is not great – It's all on a continuum.

Helping the Graded Motor Imagery process with stories and metaphors   www.noigroup.com

GMI
hand
book

C 4

106

www.noigroup.com

Helping the Graded Motor Imagery process with stories and metaphors

GMI
hand
book

3.2 CHALLENGE UNHELPFUL METAPHORS DURING THE GMI PROCESS

There are many sayings, usually metaphors which have been around for a long time. Some could now be considered unhelpful and have been proven wrong in the light of the neuroscience revolution and they should be challenged. They may well be getting in the way of your recovery. *'A little learning is a dangerous thing'* and *'ignorance is bliss'* in most circumstances should be consigned to the dustbin. This is certainly the case if you are trying to treat a chronic pain state where knowledge can be liberating. *'Time heals all wounds'* needs a challenge too. It doesn't. Time may place them in different contexts, but why would a person completely forget some of the challenges and wounds of life. *'The body is a machine'* is also problematical for most people on a GMI programme. The body is much more complex and changeable than any machine and replacing bits as you would do with a machine usually does not help with neuropathic pain.

The older members of society have many unhelpful metaphors to contend with. Next time you think a knee pain is *'just old age'* ask yourself if that knee is older than the one next to it. The aged often miss out on adequate pain treatment due to this metaphor. Our brains change right till the last breath and the saying that *'you can't teach an old dog new tricks'* is simply bullshit. We can learn to the last breath. Another widely used metaphor is *'pain is inevitable, suffering is optional'* – this needs a closer look. Pain is not an inevitable consequence of disease and injury – we all know people who have had serious injury or disease and had no pain. Is suffering optional? This could be challenged also.

Another metaphor which is erroneous is *'pain signals'* or *'pain messages'*. This is an example of an ontological metaphor where the abstract (pain) has been linked with something more concrete like a signal. But it is biologically bankrupt. There are no pain signals – our injured parts send *'danger signals'* up to the brain which then, considering all other available information, may or may not construct pain. A problem with the *'pain signals'* and *'pain messages'* metaphors is that they infer that pain comes from the tissues, whereas it comes from the brain[1].

3.3 BE A BIT PHILOSOPHICAL

When you have a pain problem for a while, you are likely to ponder the meaning of life: 'why me?' for example. In fact many people look for learning from their pain experience, or think 'it must be teaching me something'. Here are some quotes and sayings which are more in the philosophical realm and are worth pondering. *'Pain is a defender not an offender'* can be a bit difficult when you are really suffering, but pain really functions as a defender. Your brain has decided when it has weighed your world up, that you need defending and pain is one of the easiest things it can produce to defend you and make you change what you are doing. The quote should entice sufferers and clinicians alike to try to work out what threats and challenges are present to create such a defence.

'Pain is an output of the brain'. A lot of health professionals still have trouble with this one. It is so intuitive to think of pain as an input. If you pinch yourself it hurts at the site of the pinch and of course it seems like an input. But if it

was an input, it would be so easy to treat – you could stop the input by changing behaviour or taking a drug, having an injection, rubbing it, bandaging it etc. However one in four people in the world have a pain that goes on and on, so all these 'input therapies' really can't be that effective. Biologically, pain is an output like love and jealousy! And when you can take this on, it makes you engage the brain, all the things in the brain and those which can influence it.

When you have a chronic pain state it can engulf you, take over your world and everything revolves around your pain. But remembering that *'you are not your thoughts'*, as expressed so well by Eckhart Tolle[9] and Jamie Catto www.noigroup.com/videos can be very helpful. Your brain capacity is so massive and changeable (see the 'majesty of the brain' below), it has so much more spare capability than what is used to process the pain state. It says that you have the capacity to get on top of this. Catto also made another comment *'ships are safest in the harbour but that is not what they are designed for'*. We naturally retract in chronic pain states, but our coping systems are designed to explore, challenge, sniff out, engage. Let your ships venture out to sea.

John Steinbeck wrote *'one can find so many pains when the rain is falling'*. Sure, the damp weather may lead to a few more aches and pains, but Steinbeck is surely referring to the power of the brain to produce pain when the context changes – the damp weather may be one context, but time, place, mood and circumstance are others.

One of the most common metaphors that people use is *'my back (or neck or arm) is killing me.'* If you reflect on this metaphor it infers that the back is not a part of the person, but 'me' and 'the back' are two different entities. It does suggest something of an unhelpful split between brain and body. You are your body! Are you using metaphors that repeatedly separate your body from the essence of you (e.g. *'my heart is not in it'*, *'the hand is stuffed'*)?

3.4 QUOTES FROM THE FAMOUS TO KEEP YOU GOING

The GMI process and your pain state if you are a patient, can sometimes be a bit of a drag. There are many quotes around from famous and sometimes infamous people that can be useful, especially if you can relate to that famous person. The model Rachel Hunter while advertising the benefits of a new hair shampoo said *'it didn't happen overnight but it will happen'*. Patience and persistence is certainly a requirement for the best GMI outcome. The basketballer Michael Jordan famously said *'I can accept failure, everybody fails at something, but I can't accept not trying'*. This is a great quote and we are quite aware that GMI may not work for some people, but at the least we ask you to give it a good go. There are a lot of small pieces to conquer with the graded imagery programme, especially if this also entails graded exposure. Henry Ford did rather well with his car empire – he would say *'nothing is particularly hard if you divide it into small parts'*. That is what we are doing with the graded exposure strategies in GMI.

C 4

108

www.noigroup.com

Helping the Graded Motor Imagery process with stories and metaphors

GMI
hand
book

Vince Lombardi is a well known American football coach. He had some great inspirational sayings such as *'once you learn to quit it becomes a habit'* and *'it's not whether you get knocked down its whether you get up'*. With care, these may be useful if you are struggling with the programme. Keeping quotes local is probably a good idea. Our New Zealand friends all know that Sir Edmund Hillary, the first man to climb Mount Everest said after the event *'we knocked the bastard off'*. Some may respond to *'let's knock the bastard off'* in regard to their pain or disability state. While on Hillary, he also said *'it's not the mountain that we conquer but ourselves'*.

Sometimes the famous remind us of the power of changing context. Bob Marley said *'One good thing about music, when it hits you, you feel no pain'*. Jerry Lewis said a similar thing. *'When I was onstage, adrenaline killed the pain. I never hurt in front of an audience'*. Try movements and GMI components in as many different contexts as you can.

Have you got a quote that has helped you through? – you can help others by submitting it to the 'out of the shadows learning' via the contact us chapter 5, 6.2. It doesn't have to be from someone famous – it could be something your grandmother said, or even better, something that you have constructed which has helped your deep learning about GMI. Nike uses *'just do it'* of course – we think that is great for GMI, as long as you do it with as much knowledge about the process as you can gain.

4. THREE COMMON QUESTIONS ANSWERED

I have selected 3 questions that patients with chronic pain often ask and I have tried to answer them as best I can. There are many expanded metaphors in these stories and especially in the last narrative on 'the drug cabinet in the brain' see section 4.4.

4.1 WHY DON'T SOME PEOPLE BELIEVE ME?

It is likely that some people who are using the GMI programme for a chronic pain problem have been told by health professionals that 'we can't find a problem' (or inferred) that 'it is in your head' or 'I can't help you'. We think that it is very important to understand why this happens. There are a number of reasons.

The first one is that some health professionals are simply not up to date. We have made the statement in this GMI Handbook that we know more about pain in the last 10 years than in the thousand years before. One issue which many health professionals have been reluctant to take on is central sensitisation. Peripheral sensitisation is when inflammation and physical forces sensitise tissues and peripheral nerves. Central sensitisation is defined as 'amplification of neural signalling within the central nervous system that elicits pain hypersensitivity'[12]. It often coexists with peripheral sensitisation, though not necessarily.

Clifford Woolf, a leading researcher in the area of central sensitisation, considers that physicians who believe that people presenting with pain in the absence of pathology are either seeking work/insurance related compensation, are opioid drug users or suffer psychiatric disorders, may well be wrong.

Central changes, or brain and spinal cord changes are real, can be 'seen' experimentally on a brain scan, are very common and can be managed. Central mechanisms explain many pain states and provide a biological target for treatments such as graded motored imagery. It is not only physicians who may not be up to date, due to the speed of pain associated neuroscience, we would say that all professions in rehabilitation will have members with knowledge gaps. Admittedly it can be hard to keep up but education is now available.

The second and linked reason is the prevalence of biomedical thinking in health. Biomedical thinking is intuitive and it relates to the 'find the injury, the fracture, the bacteria, the virus and fix it' thinking. This can work extremely well of course and some readers may be alive today because of such thinking. But the 'find the cause and fix it' does not work so well with chronic problems where there are multiple causes and the problems are often more related to what a person thinks, knows and does about the problem. In this situation, biopsychosocial thinking, an approach that absorbs the relevant biomedical aspects, expands them to include the brain and integrates them with psychological and social issues, works better. For those interested, the following references will provide more reading on this issue[4,5,11].

The final reason, and linked with the two above, is what is known as the mind/body split or even brain/body split. This is still widely held in society and it means that the mind (or sometimes brain) is considered separate to the body. It is often referred to as Cartesian dualism, (perhaps unfairly) after the French philosopher Rene Descartes who described sensation and pain as a body event AND a mind event. There are plenty of examples in society, such as two medical professions dealing with neurones – neurology (body) and psychiatry (mind) or perhaps you have been told that if it can't be found in your body, it is in your mind. Even the terms 'physical exercise' and physical rehabilitation are fundamentally wrong – they deny the role of the brain[10]. Many pain sufferers have been a victim of this split and the results can be quite cruel. Our view is that such a hard division between mind and body is wrong and it denies the great unity between the two – of course what you think can influence your body and what you do with your body can influence your mind.

So let's put Rene Descartes in the bin and move on. It may mean that some people in pain may have to forgive some of actions of the health professionals they have seen in the past. This is important for you to take control as with this manual you are very likely to acquire more knowledge about your problem than many health professionals will have.

C 4

110

www.noigroup.com
Helping the Graded Motor Imagery process with stories and metaphors

GMI
hand
book

4.2   HOW DOES THE BRAIN WORK?

I wish we knew the answer, but maybe it's best we don't! We do know lots about parts of the brain but not so much about how it is put together to create things like consciousness and pain. One thing is for sure – the brain is the principal target organ of GMI. In this section I want to add to Lorimer's chapter and present something of the majesty of the brain, and discuss again the neuromatrix, neurosignatures and neurotags.

4.2.1 The majesty of the brain

The brain is a far more exciting organ to treat than a muscle or a ligament. Living brains are warm, a creamy colour, soft like a ripe brie cheese and move around a bit when you wriggle your head. A brain weighs around 1.5kg and is beautifully protected by the skull and some of the strongest ligaments in the body, all of which underscore how important the brain is. There are around 100 billion neurones and at least ten times as many glial cells. Glial cells can produce immune compounds, so we should say that the brain is a neuroimmune organ. This is important because some of changes in the brain in chronic pain which are targets of GMI are due to immune responses.

All these cells in your brain adore blood. Brains are about 2% of body weight but they will take 25% of the oxygen in every heartbeat. The estimated number of patterns that neurones in the brain could form with other nerve cells is 1 followed by 800 zeroes! That is heaps – more than the number of particles in the universe. Einstein would have had around the same number of neurones as you the

reader but perhaps he had a greater density of connections in some of the areas used in mathematics. In some people suffering chronic pain, pain 'becomes' them and all they observe in themselves is pain and they construct a life around that pain. Yet the story of brain biology tells us that our brains have an enormous capacity which is much bigger than one series of thoughts such as pain. For some, this may allow you to see your life from a more positive perspective. Reflect here on Tolle's statement earlier – *'you are not your thoughts'*. Or as one sufferer commented *'I can find a space in my brain for pain and put it there'*.

The exceptional feature of this organ is its changeability or plasticity. Our brains won't stop changing until we die. Change can happen in a number of ways. Making and losing synapses is one way. Children make and lose millions of synapses a second, adolescents lose 25,000 synapses a second in their visual areas. It can also quickly change to another neurosignature – from pain to no pain, from pleasure to pain, from happy to sad.

A different way to look at your brain is that its real power is to dampen things down – it is a powerful inhibitor as well as a creator of extraordinary and varied outputs. Sometimes people with head injuries can't dampen messages to muscles and spasticity occurs. There are far more neurones going down your spinal cord than coming up. People in chronic pain need a dampening down (reinhibition) of some brain areas and this is one aim of graded motor imagery and the associated education strategies.

This changeability is important for you to be aware off. These days we say the brain is not 'hard wired', it is more 'soft wired' and this means that it is much easier to change. But when you reflect on the metaphors people often use to describe their brains, they are quite mechanical (*'it's a bit rusty in there'; 'my brain is ticking'; 'got to get the cogs turning'*) and it downplays the power and potential of change. We need more up to date metaphors such as *'my synapses are fizzing' 'the networks are alive', 'my dendrites are dancing'* – whatever!

If you are interested in this area then it is worth reading more. A great read is Norman Doidge's 'The Brain that Changes Itself'[2]. It should give hope and lift your level of outcome expectation.

4.2.2 The neuromatrix, neurosignatures and neurotags

Here are a few new words! We have been using them a bit throughout the handbook and I want to briefly bring them up again. We love these words. The *neuromatrix* is a newish term for what psychologists used to call the 'coding space' of the brain. This is every possible connection in the brain. But don't think of it as 'hard wired' because this coding space is changing all the time as glial cells and synapses change activity. A neurosignature (or we call it a neurotag, like a graffiti tag[1]) is a pattern of activity in the neuromatrix. It is a physical linking of neurones at a particular time and it can lead to an output such as pain, movement or an emotion. We are not conscious of most of these brain constructions and their outputs, but rest assured that it will be a pain neurosignature, absolutely personalised for you that will be the basis behind you experience of pain (Figure 4.3).

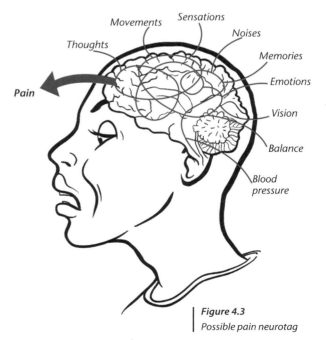

Figure 4.3
Possible pain neurotag

Pain

Thoughts
Movements
Sensations
Noises
Memories
Emotions
Vision
Balance
Blood pressure

Remember pin screens? (Figure 4.4) They were actually quite trendy in the 80s and everyone wanted one but they were usually broken at parties. Imagine the board represents all the nerve cells in the brain, although in reality each pin would represent about half a billion neurones. If I press my hand onto the pinscreen, the pins representing my fingers in my brain are activated. These nerve cells and the relationship between them are my hand neurotag. Note that they are delineated – the nails outside the fingers are not in action so the finger is given clear definition. We do know however that in some chronic pain states, there is no longer a clear and definable hand in the brain and that when the hand is touched or moved instead of a clear hand in the brain, previously pins which were non-members of the hand neurotag are now activated. It's as if you were pressing on the pinscreen with a hand covered in mud or concrete. The component therapies in GMI aim to restore the clear hand neurotag in the brain.

This activation of the 'hand' pins (nerve cells) in the brain is just one part of a possible pain neurotag. Pain neurotags could have hundreds of different parts in action linking up at any one time – so many things can influence your pain. It can be turned up and ready to fire when you are expecting pain and it can be turned off by distraction or change of context. Tim has written about changing pain neurotags with the components of the GMI package, but knowledge will also change the firing of a pain neurotag. Think of the pain you may have, which can decrease with the knowledge that you have a doctor's appointment and which may decrease even more when you have the knowledge that not much is wrong with you.

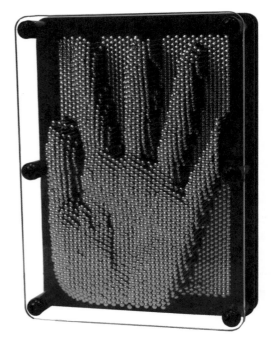

Figure 4.4 A hand
neurotag on a pin screen

4.3   WHY DO WE HURT?

We can talk about pain neurotags, but it doesn't fully answer the question of why we hurt. This topic has concerned, entertained and attracted thought and argument from the worlds of science, philosophy and the streets. Most people and many textbooks will say we hurt to be warned of impending danger or because you have taken things too far. To some degree this is true. However it is really worth going a little deeper. As a warning system it can fail us – we don't have pain when there is carbon monoxide about and we are not painfully warned of many slow growing tumours until too late, so as a warning system it has a few faults. Perhaps a deeper reason is that pain is something that makes us change behaviour or perhaps think about our behaviour, all with the goal of defending us. There is no doubt that pain is often effective in making us change behaviour, especially behaviour related to acute injury. But if you, the reader are sitting there, uncomfortable and experiencing pain that has continued for some time, you are absolutely right to ask *'what behaviour is it trying to make me change?'* and perhaps you might say *'that doesn't quite make sense in my case.'*

The angle we take here, first and foremost is that pain is absolutely real. If you say 'it hurts', you are the only witness and therefore it hurts. Secondly, this thing pain that your brain has made is essentially a defender, trying to look after you. This may be hard to reason when you are in severe pain, but even so, you created it from within because your brain, pulling together all the information it has to hand from within and around your body, has calculated that your body, your 'self', has something about it that needs defending. This is quite obvious in the case of a sprained ankle. However, in more longstanding situations, the information that your brain uses to make the decision to create pain comes from many sources such as your knowledge, what you have been told, your thoughts and beliefs, emotions, your needs, your concepts and your memories.

Sometimes the question we could equally ask is – *'why do we not hurt'*. To help answer this question, let's look at the remarkable story of the drug cabinet in the brain.

4.4 POWERFUL NATURAL DRUGS IN OUR BRAINS – OUR OWN DRUG CABINET

Deep in our brains, between the tops of our ears, are brain areas which work together (so, a neurotag) to produce some very powerful painkillers. (The names of these parts include the periaqueductal gray and the rostroventral medulla – but don't worry – many clinicians may not even know these names). This area is what I call the personal drug cabinet of the brain (Figure 4.5). We all have one. Unfortunately, this drug cabinet has been somewhat hijacked by the commercial drug companies. Ask yourself to name four or more painkillers readily available from the pharmacy: Easy! Panadol, Aspirin, Advil and Nurofen. But we have trouble naming four that our own brain makes such as serotonin, and the opioids such as enkephalins, endorphins and even morphine. These are the HHs (Happy hormones in my sketch). And by the way, yours are free and potentially more powerful than the man-made ones. There are no side effects and no need for a prescription either.

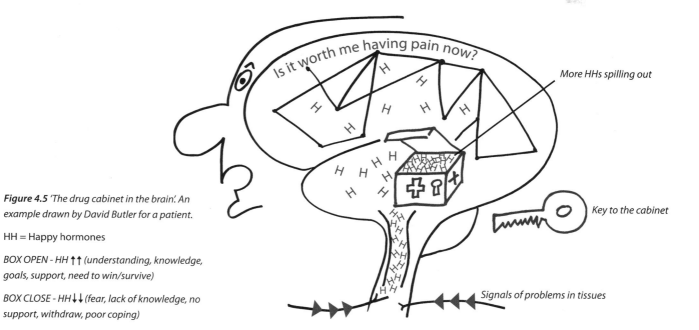

Figure 4.5 'The drug cabinet in the brain'. An example drawn by David Butler for a patient.

HH = Happy hormones

BOX OPEN - HH ↑↑ (understanding, knowledge, goals, support, need to win/survive)

BOX CLOSE - HH↓↓ (fear, lack of knowledge, no support, withdraw, poor coping)

4.4.1 The cabinet

When scientists electrically zap the drug cabinet area in a rat's brain, you can stop what appears to be rat pain[8]. The zapping turns on the internal painkillers. This was tried out on humans with limited success as unfortunately it also creates awful migraines, so zapping it isn't the best way to get into the cabinet. There are other ways.

If you think about it, it should be quite obvious that our body has a way of controlling pain – either turning it up or turning it down. Perhaps readers have a memory of having had an injury but no pain – or most likely you have read about a similar situation in the papers. Perhaps a sportsman has finished a game and complained of no pain yet has a severe injury such as a fracture (See also chapter 1 of *Explain Pain*).

One of the reasons we make our own painkillers is that it allows us to survive and do things when we have to. There are many stories about people who have had nasty accidents on a farm when they are alone, but have said that there was no pain. This does make sense – what use is pain when you are on your own without anyone to listen to your complaints? Best to put survival resources into shock or movement. And you certainly don't need any more warning. Pain can wait a bit, often until when you can see a health professional. It's safe to have pain then!

4.4.2 The power of your drug cabinet

Have no doubt about the power of your drug cabinet in your brain. Some people have estimated that it can be up to 50 times more powerful than any drug man has ever invented. Wow! If you think of those stories above where people have had horrible injury but no pain it tells us that this system is really powerful. For every neurone in your nervous system that could influence pain going up to your brain there are 200 coming down. You should also know that it is highly sophisticated. Many drugs combine together very smoothly to stop pain. When man made drugs get mixed up, there are often complications.

And by the way, for any drug you buy to actually work it has to 'turn on' your own pain killing system in your brain.

You could ask 'if it is so powerful why can't I use it all the time'. Of course, the synthetic pain medications and anti-inflammatories are very welcome, they are improving, and we should be grateful for them. But they work best when there is acute pain and inflammation, far better than in chronic pain states when tissues have had plenty of time to heal. If you are a patient using GMI, it is likely that the man-made drugs will have little or no effect on your pain.

4.4.3 How does the drug cabinet work?

From the drug cabinet, (Figure 4.5) your internal morphine like chemicals (the HHs) are released both into the brain and into the spinal cord where they can limit or even stop impulses coming in from body structures. This remarkable drug cabinet can also turn up the impulses coming into the spinal cord, simply by lessening the amount of your painkillers. Note how there is a supercontrol system. Just like governments usually regulate what kinds of drugs are sold, your higher brain can regulate which drugs your body needs. But your higher brain has a job to do here and it basically has to answer the question *'is it really worth me having pain now'*. This is the ultimate question the brain considers when deciding how much morphine-like substances to let out of the drug cabinet. In Figure 4.5, some of the issues the brain has to consider to work this out are listed. They include anticipating pain (cabinet closes = less painkillers) memories of previous pains (cabinet may close), pain not desirable at this time – need to survive or win the grand final (cabinet opens = more painkillers), in a dangerous situation (cabinet closes), everything is OK – life is cruisy (cabinet opens).

So there is a key to the drug cabinet. To turn it off and dry up the pain killers you need to be concerned, worried about reinjury, have no goals, focus on every little thing, be angry, avoid learning about your problems and withdraw from life and movement.

To open it up and dribble the painkillers down through the spinal cord and brain, you need to be basically OK with your lot in life, have knowledge and understanding, be aware of coping and treatment strategies, and have support to utilise. But basically, knowledge is the greatest pain liberator of all.

The key is in your hands.

REFERENCES

1. Butler DS, Moseley GL. *Explain Pain*. Adelaide: NOI Publications, 2003.

2. Doidge N. *The brain that changes itself*. Viking Press, New York, 2008.

3. Gallagher L, McAuley J, Moseley, GL. A randomised controlled trial of using a book of metaphors to reconceptualise pain and decrease catastrophising in people with chronic pain. *Clinical Journal of Pain* (in press) 2012.

4. Gatchel RJ, Peng YB, Peters ML, et al. The biopsychosocial approach to chronic pain: Scientific advances and future directions. *Psychological Bulletin* 2007;133:581-624.

5. Jones M, Edwards I, Gifford LS. A conceptual model for the implementation of biopsychosocial therapy in clinical practice *Manual Therapy* 2000;7:2-9.

6. Lakoff G, Johnson M. *Metaphors we live by*. Chicago: University of Chicago Press, 1980.

7. Moseley GL. *Painful Yarns. Metaphors and stories to help understand the biology of pain*. Canberra: Dancing Giraffe Press, 2008.

8. Reynolds DV. Surgery in the rat during electrical analgesia induced by focal brain stimulation. *Science* 1969;154:444-5.

9. Tolle E. *The Power of Now: A guide to spiritual enlightenment*. New World Library, Novato, 2005.

10. Wade D. Why physical medicine, physical disability and physical rehabilitation? We should abandon Cartesian dualism. *Clin Rehab* 2006;20:85-90.

11. Weiner BK. Spine update: The biopsychosocial model and spine care. *Spine* 2008;33:219-23.

12. Woolf CJ. Central sensitization: Implications for the diagnosis and treatment of pain. *Pain* 2011;152:S2-15.

NOTES

The Graded Motor Imagery toolbox
Thomas J. Giles

1. PATIENCE, PERSISTENCE, COURAGE AND COMMITMENT

My older brother and I saved our pocket money for months to buy our first skateboard when I was three. This would see me rolling for years to come. At high school I went into a skateboarding phase and still haven't quite come out of it. Without a car as transport, skating was about rolling around the smoothest parts of the neighbourhood looking for things to 'grind', 'ollie' or go really 'fast down'.

Tricks like 'ollies', 'manuals', 'grinds', 'boardslides' and 'kickflips' were what defined skating for me as a young teenager and I spent all my spare time trying to learn the tricks which a few of my skatie mates had mastered. See Box 5.1

I had a few of these tricks down but was keen to master the kickflip which, if I ever tried, would make me feel like I had slow legs, uncoordinated feet and no strength. With the persistence of a stubborn teenager I was committed to master the 'kickflip' and thus began the countless hours of practising each day after school. After weeks, months and plenty of gravel rashes I remember walking in one night as Dad was serving up a delicious pasta I blurted out *'I give up!'* Hot, sweaty and exhausted I had gone to the world's end to try to do a 'stupid' kickflip.

I was clearly shooting past my skill level and with the help of some bolognaise I realised that I had to take some steps back. Like learning an instrument or language, I slowed the process down and broke it up – paying attention to ollies and balance (manuals) instead. These skills needed to be honed before I would have a chance of busting out a kickflip 'on the go'. Time passed and a year later I could sometimes pull one off while becoming a master at the ollie and manual! Patience and persistence, courage, commitment and confidence were key.

I'm not a physio (thankfully, this book needs some variety!). I'm the office nerd, the email guy, they call me the 'Recognise man'. When I read the chapters from Lorimer, Tim and David before, it became clear that the mastery of the skateboard is in my brain too and to some degree it's not that much different to getting the best out of graded motor imagery.

Like skateboarding, GMI is not a quick and easy process but hopefully with the tools I will be introducing to you in this chapter you can explore the various levels of brain exercises out there and achieve pain relief and better function.

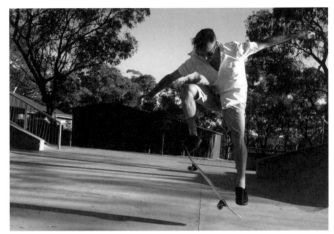

Figure 5.1A Tom in the skatepark popping an Ollie

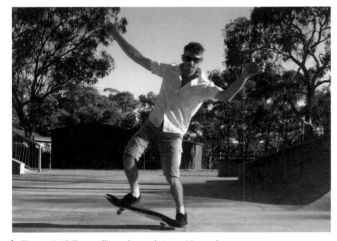

Figure 5.1B Tom rolling along, doing a Manual

Box 5.1 For the uninitiated

Ollie: popping the board in the air, or jumping. This is done by pushing down with your back foot and jumping up leading with your front foot to 'balance' the board and raise the back. Getting air! (Figure 5.1A).

Manual: Rolling along with the front two wheels off the ground without letting the rear tail touch the ground. Getting around and staying balanced on your back two wheels. (Figure 5.1B).

Grind: This generally requires an 'ollie' onto a smooth, thin surface such as a railing, kerb, bench, etc. with the aim of sliding along on the trucks (axle), not the wheels or board.

Boardslide: same as a grind except using the bit of board between the trucks to slide along the surface.

Kickflip: This is similar to an ollie, but instead of just leading the jump with the front foot – you flick the board with the ball of your foot to make it spin underneath you while in the air. So you land it wheels down. Tricky stuff!

2.   THE GMI TOOLBOX

There are a number of tools currently available for GMI.

Recognise is a comprehensive online left/right discrimination tool built for implicit (exercising your brain without realising you are) and explicit (more intentional) motor imagery exercises.

Recognise Flash Cards are a set of 48 'vanilla' (plain background) images, like a set of cards, built to train your left/right discrimination. These complement the online programme and are particularly useful if you are on the move and/or don't have computer access.

Recognise App is another left/right discrimination tool which you can keep in your pocket. With most modern phones or devices you can now do your brain training exercises anywhere.

Mirrors NOI's mirror box is suitable for use for the upper limb and feet. If needed, larger mirror boxes are easy enough to construct yourself.

Other Do It Yourselfs include magazines, photos from the internet or your personal photos, and the power of imagination.

Each of these tools is now discussed in detail.

3.   RECOGNISE

3.1   SYSTEM REQUIREMENTS

Recognise is an online computer programme which you can use to assess and treat your left/right discrimination abilities. It is the most comprehensive tool available for motor imagery exercises. With this tool you can 'put your lefts and rights back in your brain'. With a computer and an internet connection anywhere in the world, you can do your exercises, keep an eye on your progression with all of your results and connect with a clinician for further guidance.

You'll be glad to know you don't need to be a geek to make sure Recognise works on your computer, but you will require:

- A reasonably modern computer and screen (desktop, laptop or tablet)
- An internet connection (dial up is too slow)
- A keyboard
- An email address

Recognise also works on other new fancy devices like the iPad. Don't stress! Like all things such as skateboarding it's easy once you know how – so I'll now take you through setting up a new Recognise account and get started using actual 'screen grabs' from the programme.

C 5

1 2 5

The Graded Motor Imagery toolbox
www.noigroup.com

GMI
hand
book

3.2 STARTING UP A RECOGNISE ACCOUNT

If you're using Recognise you'll need to have your own account. If you don't already have one, go to www.noigroup.com/recognise to buy a two month account or set up a free trial account. Your screen will look like Figure 5.3. There is heaps of information about Recognise on this page.

Once you've set up your Recognise account as a full account or trial you can start straight away if you know what you're doing. Use your initial tests to construct a baseline score of your current left/right discrimination capacity, then decide where to go from here:

A. Continue with left/right discrimination exercises, customising them as necessary.

B. Or move along the sequential process to imagined movements or mirrors (this may be appropriate for more acute pain states as discussed in chapter 3).

Your clinician will be very helpful here and so will Tim's chapter. These trial test results will give you an indication of whether there is a laterality deficit as part of your problem. All results are kept in your Recognise account from day one. You can view these results on a graph for comparison and progression once you've done a few tests, but we'll discuss this later.

As a GMI user there are two styles of Recognise accounts – **patients** and **clinicians**. Both are similar, but there are important differences you should know about, depending on who you are and your role in using Recognise. Let's look at this from the patient's perspective first.

GMI hand book

Figure 5.2A
Recognise homescreen

C 5

1 2 7

Recognise: left/right discrimination, recognition and restoration

Recognise is the first way to accurately measure the ability to recognise left and right body parts and movement, and to train left/right discrimination as part of a comprehensive rehabilitation programme.

The ability to recognise a part of the body as belonging or moving to the left or the right involves brain processes that are important for normal function. In some situations, for example after injury, the ability to recognise body parts and movements as being left or right becomes reduced. Sometimes, the ability to recognise whether a body part is moving to the left or the right becomes reduced. These problems may contribute to pain and loss of function. Getting better at recognising left and right body parts and movements has been shown to reduce pain, aids recovery from injury and improves performance. Learn more...

Log in

email:

password:

☐ I agree to the terms & conditions

forgotten something?   log in

Trial

Sign up here for a free trial of 5 logins
with most features of Recognise.

Purchase

buy a full Recognise account here

Figure 5.2B
Setting up a trial account

GMI
hand
book

Recognise: left/right discrimination, recognition and restoration

Simply fill in this form to get started with your trial - this will last for five separate logins.

NOTE: if you are already a member of Noigroup you can use the same email and password to login to Recognise from the homepage.

Once your trial has expired, you can still login to access all historical results and notes.

Upgrade to a full account from the homepage to continue your exercises and keep all trial period results.

first name: *

last name: *

email: *

country: select... ⌄ *

password: *

confirm: *

time zone: select... ⌄ *

noi notes: ⦿ yes ○ no

sign me up

C 5

128

www.noigroup.com
The Graded Motor Imagery toolbox

GMI
hand
book

3.3   USING RECOGNISE AS A PATIENT

Make sure you are logged in using your personal membership email and password to access your Recognise account at www.noigroup.com/recognise. If you already have a Noigroup log in, this will also work for Recognise. Below is your Recognise homepage once you've logged in.

Once you've logged in this is your personal homepage; it is all fairly self-explanatory. Here you can:

- update your personal details

- extend your account expiry date

- connect (or disconnect) with a clinician

- change your account to a clinician's account

3.3.1 Extending your account
Each full Recognise account lasts for two months and trials last for five logins. All of your results are kept in your profile so you can upgrade to a full account or extend for two more months while maintaining all previous results. Extending your account can be done by you or your clinician (if you and your clinician are 'connected' but read on for more information) in further multiples of two months. Choose the number of months you expect to be using Recognise for and follow the prompts to the checkout.

3.3.2 Connect with a clinician
Connecting with your clinician will enable him or her to access and translate your results, and then suggest the best course of action. Your clinician may have recommended that you set up a Recognise account or even done it for you. Connecting on Recognise is easy, provided you know your therapist's Clinician ID and name.

We recommend that any GMI user works alongside a clinician. If your clinician, let's say it's Tim, is already on Recognise then he should have a 'Clinician ID'. If your clinician hasn't set up your account (this would imply you are already connected) and has his own Recognise clinician's account, you can connect with Tim in the system if you know his Recognise Clinician ID and full name. Follow these instructions and screens to connect with your clinician

- Go to 'connect with my clinician'

- Enter your clinician's ID

- Select your clinician from results. This will send a note to your clinician which he will see next time he accesses his Recognise account. Once your clinician confirms your request you will be connected.

3.3.3 Change to a clinician's account
If you are using Recognise as a clinician with your patient(s), you may want to change your account features. Switching to a clinician's account is free and you will be able to store and create accounts and trials to set your patients up on Recognise, and with their permission, have access to results. Obviously this isn't helpful if you are a patient, so only clinicians should do this.

3.3.4 The Graded Motor Imagery noticeboard

The Recognise noticeboard is an up-to-date resource where you will find information relating to current GMI practice and other relevant resources. All resources found on the noticeboard are archived in the Research and Literature section found in the footer of each page.

C 5

129

The Graded Motor Imagery toolbox
www.noigroup.com

GMI
hand
book

Recognise: left/right discrimination, recognition and restoration

recognise
results
notes
account
my images
log out

Welcome Lisa!
Lisa Smith
lisa@lisasmith.com
Australia
South Australia
6:54pm

Account type: Individual
First log in: 15 March 2011
Expiry: 15 May 2 011
Cinician: Lisa Smith

/Edit details

/Edit email and password

*changing details here will
change the details of your
Noigroup account*

Extend my account
Set up your account to keep doing left/right exercises for the number of months selected below. You don't need to wait until your account has expired to extend.

months [2 ▾] = $10.00 AUD [checkout]

Connect with a clinician
If your clinician has a Recognise account, enter their clinician's details below to get connected and allow your clinician access to your results. All your personal information (expect name and email) and any 'notes' will remail private. Your clinician's ID will be in a **AA1234** format.

[   ] [find]

Change to clinician's account
If you are a clinician using Recognise as a treatment tool with patients, convert your account into a clinician's account to get the most out of Recognise in your professional patient relationships. NOI recommends patients do not convert their accounts, although it won't affect your testing and results.

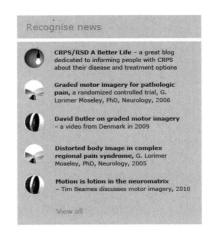

Figure 5.3
Your Recognise homepage
as a patient.

C 5

130

www.noigroup.com
The Graded Motor Imagery toolbox

GMI
hand
book

3.4   USING RECOGNISE AS A CLINICIAN

With a clinician's account you will find most parts of Recognise are the same as they are for a patient, such as your personal information, extending your account and accessing the noticeboard. All personal testing and results features within your own account will also be identical. The main difference here is you can set up or extend your patients' accounts from within your own account, and where you have permission, log in to check up on their results and progression.

3.4.1 Setting up a clinician's account

Setting up a clinician's account is free and means your account features will change. You will be able to create full accounts and trials to set your patients up to use Recognise. This isn't helpful if you are a patient, but if you are a clinician expecting to be using Recognise with even one patient (but certainly with more) you may as well adapt your account. See the previous screen grab (Figure 5.3) for where you can change your account to become a clinician.

3.4.2 Connect with your patient

To connect with your patient, let's call her Jane, you will need the name and email address which she uses for Recognise. Follow the instructions below:

- Enter patient email in 'connect with a patient'

- Confirm your patient from the list of results. This will send a request to your patient which he/she will see next time they access their Recognise account.

- Once the request is approved you will have full access to your patient's results.

3.4.3 Set up or extend your patient's account

A Starter Account sets a new patient up (or extends an existing patient's trial account) for two months access to Recognise gives you a two month account to set a patient up with Recognise or to upgrade a patient from a trial. A Starter Account can also be used to extend a patient's account for a further two months. These can alternatively be purchased by patients from the Recognise home page and www.noigroup.com/en/Category/BT. We won't go into currencies here but one of these Starter Accounts costs about the same price as a decent pizza.

Recognise: left/right discrimination, recognition and restoration

recognise
results
notes
account
my images
clinician
log out

Welcome Tom!

Tom Giles
Neuro Orthopaedic Institute
tom@noigroup.com
Australia
South Australia

Account Type: Clinician
First logged in: 11 March 2011
Expiry: 15 May 2013
Clinician number: TG0001

/Edit details

/Edit email and password

/Manage patients

*changing details here will
change the details of your
Noigroup account*

Connect with a patient

Connect with your patients to get the most out of Recognise.
Once permission is granted, you can view their test results
from your account. Patient personal details and 'notes' will
always remain private.

| enter patient email | find |

Extend my account

Extend your Recognise account at any stage by multiples of
two months to keep using the imagery exercises. You don't
have to wait for your licence to run out. If your account has
expired you no longer take tests, but can still view all results,
notes and manage patients.

months [2 ▾] = $10.00 AUD [checkout]

Buy more start-up accounts

Use start-ups to set your patients up with a 2 month account or
extend an existing patient account by any multiple of 2 months.

no. licences [1 ▾] = $20.00 AUD [checkout]

Recognise news

 CRPS/RSD A Better Life – a great blog
dedicated to informing people with CRPS
about their disease and treatment options

 **Graded motor imagery for pathologic
pain,** a randomized controlled trial, G.
Lorimer Moseley, PhD, Neurology, 2006

 David Butler on graded motor imagery
– a video from Denmark in 2009

 **Distorted body image in complex
regional pain syndrome,** G. Lorimer
Moseley, PhD, Neurology, 2005

 Motion is lotion in the neuromatrix
– Tim Beames discusses motor imagery, 2010

View all

GMI
hand
book

Figure 5.4
*Your Recognise homepage
as a clinician.*

C 5

1 3 2

www.noigroup.com
The Graded Motor Imagery toolbox

GMI
hand
book

3.5   THE LEFT/RIGHT TESTS

3.5.1 The mechanics behind the screen

Recognise has thousands of different images collected in a big pool – heads, feet, fingers, shoulders, necks etc. Each picture is randomly rotated and flipped to create eight different images. Don't worry too much about this because the computer does all the work for you here, but the point is that you won't get used to the images. Remember this if you ever think you see 'the same' image during a test… it probably isn't! Click on 'Recognise' in the top right navigation panel to start setting up a test – see Figure 5.5 here you can adjust a few variables to suit you such as time (in seconds) displayed per image and the number of images used in the test.

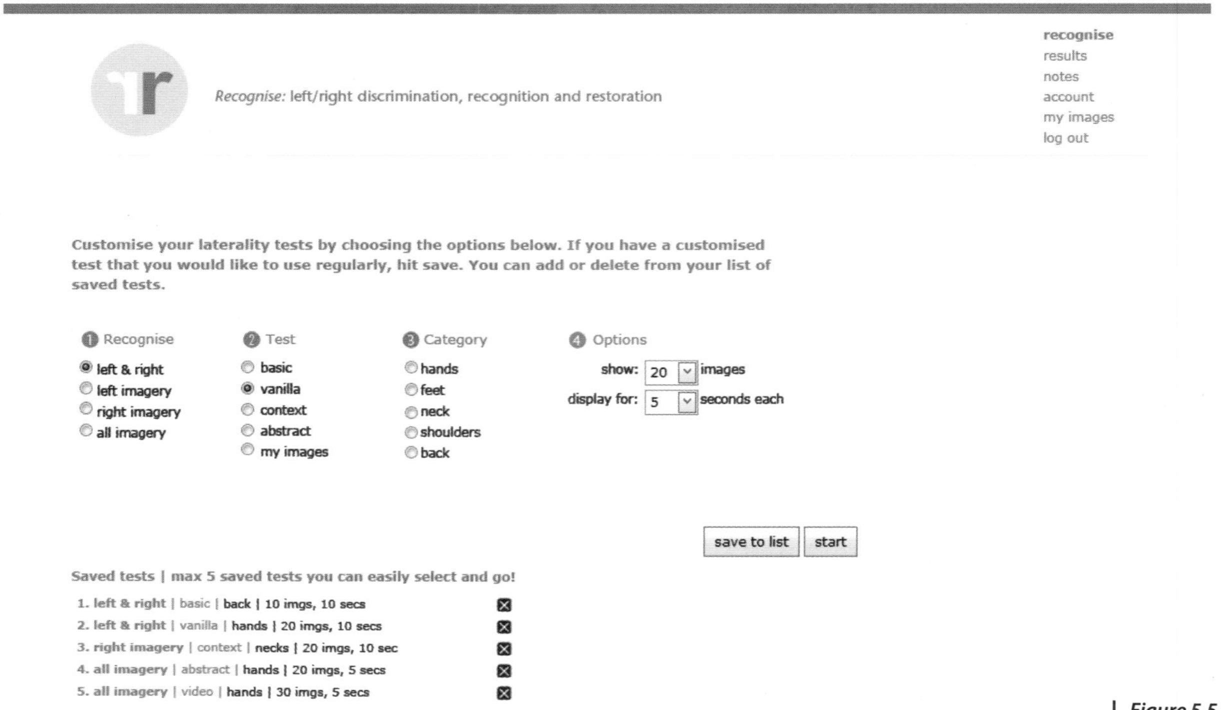

r   *Recognise:* left/right discrimination, recognition and restoration

recognise
results
notes
account
my images
log out

Customise your laterality tests by choosing the options below. If you have a customised test that you would like to use regularly, hit save. You can add or delete from your list of saved tests.

❶ Recognise

- left & right
- left imagery
- right imagery
- all imagery

❷ Test

- basic
- vanilla
- context
- abstract
- my images

❸ Category

- hands
- feet
- neck
- shoulders
- back

❹ Options

show: 20 images

display for: 5 seconds each

save to list   start

Saved tests | max 5 saved tests you can easily select and go!

1. **left & right** | basic | **back** | **10 imgs, 10 secs**   ☒
2. **left & right** | vanilla | **hands** | **20 imgs, 10 secs**   ☒
3. **right imagery** | context | **necks** | **20 imgs, 10 sec**   ☒
4. **all imagery** | abstract | **hands** | **20 imgs, 5 secs**   ☒
5. **all imagery** | video | **hands** | **30 imgs, 5 secs**   ☒

Figure 5.5 Customising and setting up your tests.

3.5.2 Customising your left/right test (Figure 5.5)

● **Recognise**

For doing a left/right recognition test you will need to select 'left & right'. The other three 'Imagery' test selections are applicable for stage two of GMI.

● **Test**

Recognise gives you a choice of basic, vanilla, context, abstract and your own images. We recommend using Recognise with pictures graded in that order as a means of grading exposure to the images.

● **Category**

Set your test up to include the body part(s) most relevant to your brain training exercise recommendations, or injury. The body parts include hands, feet, necks, shoulders, backs.

We recommend taking tests with just one body part, but you may have pain in your arm and leg which may warrant doing hands and feet together at once, or separately, as it suits you. Take this as an example and extrapolate depending on where you have pain around your body. Once again, this is an area where you may wish to consult with your clinician.

● **Options: number of images**

Our broad suggestion is to start with 20 pictures but that's a very general rule. High performance sports people may easily fly through 50 or even 100 pictures whereas others find five pictures to be a good starting point. All of these variations depend on you as the individual and need to be set at a comfortable level. Tim has some advice in his chapter about setting a baseline, but it often requires some trial and error. You may be doing these types of exercises each day for a number of weeks or months so don't wear yourself out early on. Think of it as a powerful brain retraining game with yourself.

You can choose the following number of images: 2, 4, 6, 8, 10, 12, 14, 16, 18, 20, 30, 40, 50, 60, 70, 80, 90, 100.

● **Options: time**

You can adjust the maximum time (in seconds) that each picture is displayed for until it 'times out' and moves onto the next. We generally recommend starting at 5 seconds per image and take it from there but you might prefer something faster or slower and this can be adjusted from test to test. Initially, make sure you've got more than enough time, then start pushing yourself, grading down the time per image to as quick as possible. Be careful! If an image times out and moves onto the next, it will be scored in your results as incorrect.

You can choose the following times (seconds per image): 1, 2, 3, 4, 5, 6, 7, 8, 9, 10, 20, 30.

If you're ready, go to 'start' to begin your test (Figure 5.5), you will then be asked whether you want to record your pain level.

The Graded Motor Imagery toolbox
www.noigroup.com

GMI
hand
book

GMI
hand
book

Figure 5.6B
Vanilla image

Figure 5.6C
Context image

Figure 5.6D
Abstract image

IMAGE TYPES

A basic image is one which is displayed from a natural point of view with a vanilla (consistent non-distracting) background. This image hasn't been rotated. Depending on your injury or pain level, this might be your best starting point. Using basic images means you require less brain work to determine the laterality than with a rotated (or upside down) image.

Vanilla images are the same as basic images except they are randomly rotated 90, 180 and 270 degrees. They all have a plain, mono-coloured background, so there is no distraction. Like the basic choice, this is a safe place to start although a little more difficult than the basic images.

Context images will take you to places like your home, work, the beach, colours, injury, and maybe some places you'd rather not be. Depending on the context of each image and your previous life experiences, this can make your ability to judge left or right more or less difficult as your brain has to deal with the context as well as the left/right issue. What if you broke your wrist on a building site and there were images of hands, tools and bricks? Or what if you have foot pain and were presented with a foot with 12 stitches in it? All images in Recognise have been chosen based on their everyday merits. Some of these images, particularly where injury has been displayed, may be a little shocking. If this is the case, please discuss with your clinician. See chapter 2, 5.4.1 for a patient example.

Abstract images are exactly how they sound. In this lot of images you'll find blurred pictures, shapes which imitate body parts, animal body parts, shoes, gloves, imprints, patterns and so on. These are pictures which are likely to take a bit more brain exercise to work out if they're left or right.

Recognise offers you a very powerful 'My Images' tool (Figure 5.7). You can keep a file of your own images including those of your own body parts – perhaps pre-injury or in plaster cast for example. Use up to 50 images at a time with the option to replace/update them as your left/right discrimination skills improve.

- Follow the 'my images' link on the top right of your screen to add your own images.

- Nominate the category (hands, feet, back, neck etc) of your image, then simply upload them from your computer using the 'browse' facility. You can upload ten images at once.

- When uploaded, specify whether the image is left or right by clicking the appropriate text under each one. This will activate the image. We recommend you do this with another person to make absolutely sure that you have correctly coded the images.

- Delete your images by clicking the small red x on each one.

- If your image count has reached 50 you will need to delete existing images to replace them with new ones.

GMI
hand
book

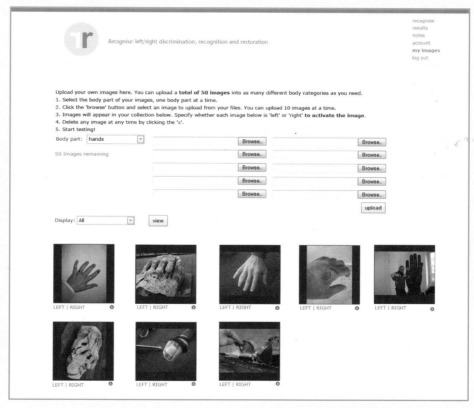

Figure 5.7 Adding your own images to Recognise

GMI
hand
book

3.5.3 Your pain level

This is a means of recording your pain level before taking each test (Figure 5.8). It is optional and any information you provide will be recorded against each test for you to observe in your results. This is handy to look back on, especially with your clinician. '0' is no pain at all, '10' is very severe pain where you would like me to call an ambulance now.

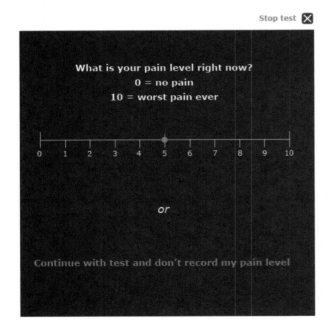

Figure 5.8 *Recording your current pain level and/or continuing with your test.*

3.6 STOP TEST!

On the top right hand side of your test screen there will always be a quick exit button called 'Stop test' (Figure 5.9). Use this if you need to stop half way through your test for whatever reason, for example, if you are disturbed from your test or in rare circumstances start feeling too distressed, uncomfortable, or too tired. The image will disappear immediately and you will be taken straight back to set up a new test (Figure 5.5). Your results from the interrupted test will not be recorded.

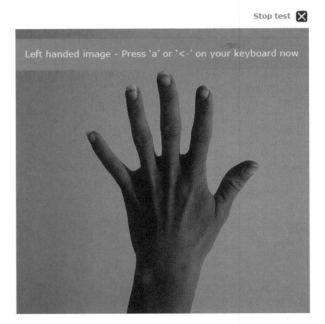

Figure 5.9
Quick exit button

3.7 TEST PERFORMANCE

When you start using Recognise make sure you are in a relaxed and quiet place. Start sitting first, but as you progress you might like to try it standing or even lying in front of the computer screen. Have your fingers ready on a 'left' and 'right' key to start. The key to signal that it is a left image on the screen is 'a' or '<'(LEFT ARROW). The key to signal that it is a right image on the screen is 'd' or '>' (RIGHT ARROW). Note that the left and right keys are close to each other so if one arm is very painful or even if you are missing an arm you can still take the test using one hand by using the index finger on one key and the middle finger on the other. However, if using the keyboard is really too difficult or uncomfortable we recommend you install voice recognition software onto your computer. Contact your local computer shop for help here.

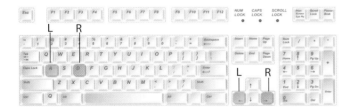

Now you're ready to go! This is where you will be presented with sample left and right images to make sure you're comfortable with the process. Try to figure out as quickly and accurately as possible whether the image on the screen is left or right and press 'left' or 'right' appropriately. After the first two images (which aren't recorded) you'll be on your way.

3.7.1 How did you go?

When you finish your test you will see the screen (Figure 5.10) which briefly summarises your results in terms of accuracy and speed. From here you can choose to either:

A. take the same test again

B. view your entire history of test results

C. set up a new test

To get a real sense of where you're at, we do recommend that the test is repeated at least three times. Current research has gathered 'normal' results for tests of different body parts. Normal results vary from body part to body part. Tim goes through what we call 'normal' results (chapter 3 Figure 3.14A-E) and Lorimer discusses some of the experiments that have allowed us to suggest these normal figures (chapter 2, section 4).

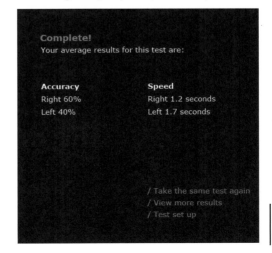

Figure 5.10
Test complete!
Results summary

C 5

1 3 7

The Graded Motor Imagery toolbox
www.noigroup.com

GMI
hand
book

3.8 TRANSLATING RESULTS

When you land on your results page (following a test or clicking 'results' on the top right menu) you will see your recent test results displayed in both graph and table form which can both be used to translate the important data (see Figure 5.11A,B).

Accuracy and speed: Results are displayed either in terms of accuracy as a percentage or speed (response time) in seconds. Click between these two variables on the y axis to see them appear in the graph, see Figure 5.11A.

Trend line: The trend line smooths out any 'off' days or uncharacteristic lumps you might have in your results.

While these off days and lumps are important to know about, the trend line is used to reveal the overall direction of progression after you've done a dozen or more tests. Your trend line should ideally go up for 'accuracy' and down for 'speed'. These are signs of progression in a positive direction. Click the trend line button 'on' or 'off' below the x-axis to view your results with or without this feature.

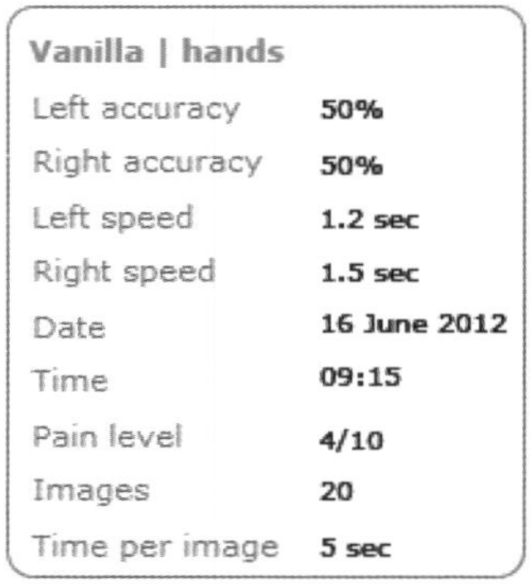

Pain level: If you've entered your pain rating before a test you will be able to see these details recorded in the side panel of your results as you click from point to point on your results graph.

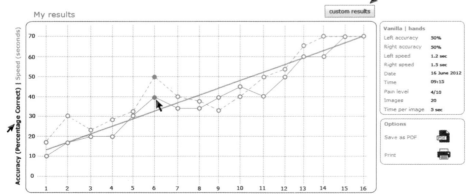

Click here to go to Figure 5.12

Details						Speed		Accuracy	
Date	Time	Test	Images	Image time	Pain level	L	R	L	R
12-Mar-2012	10:40	vanilla | hands	20	6	n/a	0.4s	0.2s	50%	50%
12-Mar-2012	10:40	vanilla | hands	15	6	7/10	0.3s	0.2s	30%	40%
10-Mar-2012	14:39	vanilla | hands	20	6	n/a	0.1s	0.1s	70%	60%
06-Mar-2012	16:59	vanilla | hands	20	5	3/10	0.4s	0.7s	100%	0%
06-Mar-2012	16:59	vanilla | hands	10	5	n/a	0.1s	0.1s	70%	50%
06-Mar-2012	16:58	vanilla | hands	20 / 10	6 / 4	6/10	0.1s	0.1s	40%	40%

Figure 5.11A
Your results page (these are not true results)

Figure 5.11B
Click on an orange or green point on the graph to recall the specific test information which is displayed in the panel above.

3.8.1 A CLOSER LOOK AT YOUR RESULTS

While the initial results summary provides you with your most recent results, you or your clinician are eventually likely to want a more detailed and historical summary. Recognise offers advanced filtering and graphic displays. Just click the 'custom results' button above your results graph to find your way there.

Date range: You may want to look up your results for last week compared to this week. To do this, select the start and end dates for the time you want to view along with which tests you want results to be displayed for and hit 'view/go'. Test type and category: Similar to setting up a test, you can define quite specifically which results you'd like to see. For example, you can look for all of the results for basic hands OR vanilla feet OR context necks and so on. Alternatively you can choose to view the results from all of your tests at once – this will depend on what questions you want to answer from the data in your results.

The custom results page allows you to find information on:

- Your most recent tests (25, 50, 100)

- Isolating specific test types

- Results from a specific date range

- Your accuracy and speed trends over time

Initially we suggest that there is no need to customise your results but as you progress and time passes, you or your clinician may want to see more specific results such as those from a certain date range or for particular body parts. Use the 'custom results' link on your results page to access the advanced filtering options in Figure 5.12.

C 5

1 3 9

www.noigroup.com

The Graded Motor Imagery toolbox

GMI
hand
book

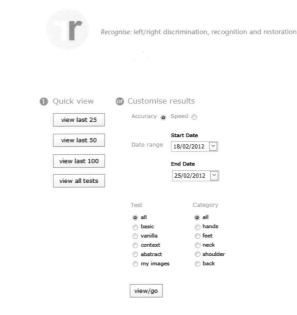

Figure 5.12 *Results – quick view and customising your results*

C 5

140

www.noigroup.com

The Graded Motor Imagery toolbox

GMI
hand
book

3.9   ADDING NOTES

Recognise is set up so you can make and keep your own notes within your account (Figure 5.13). These might be thoughts, experiences, feelings, moods or whatever you want to write down and they are completely private (your clinician can't even see them).

You may find it beneficial to read back over your notes and compare your thoughts from the past with your results from the same period. Or it may just help to relieve some stress at the time by getting your thoughts out of your head and into your notes. It might not only be your day to day experiences the notes will help you explore, there may be times when Recognise is discomforting to use or the snapshot images you go through dig up memories from the past or evoke feelings you don't want. Use this as a personal and free flowing notebook or diary.

Go to: > Notes > Create new

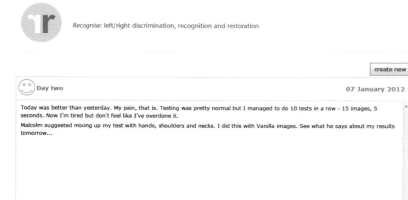

Recognise: left/right discrimination, recognition and restoration

create new

Day two   07 January 2012

Today was better than yesterday. My pain, that is. Testing was pretty normal but I managed to do 10 tests in a row - 15 images, 5 seconds. Now I'm tired but don't feel like I've overdone it.

Malcolm suggested mixing up my test with hands, shoulders and necks. I did this with Vanilla images. See what he says about my results tomorrow...

View older posts

1 january 2012	12:11	*trial*	⊠
2 february 2012	21:04	*day 1*	⊠
3 march 2012	09:45	*day 2*	⊠

***Figure 5.13** Adding notes on Recognise*

3.10 USING RECOGNISE FOR (EXPLICIT) MOTOR IMAGERY

You can also use Recognise for stage two of the step-by-step GMI process, explicit motor imagery. Explicit simply means that you're doing it on purpose; find more on this in chapter 3. These exercises are something you can begin to integrate while going on with your left/right discrimination. Using Recognise as a motor imagery tool is as easy as setting up a test (Figure 5.5). All you need to do is select 'left imagery', 'right imagery' or 'all imagery'.

3.10.1 What's the difference?

The main differences in using Recognise as an imagined movements (stage two) tool are:

- **There are no results recorded**
  This is a brain exercise which requires no feedback, just practice, mental exercises and repetition. No results are recorded but you still might want to make some personal notes in your account.

- **Choose 'left only', 'right only' or 'left and right' images**
  Take time to do motor imagery exercises for each side, but we recommend paying most attention to your affected side.

- **Each image to be displayed for 10, 20 or 30 seconds**
  Use this time frame to mentally run through the position/movement and any related sensation such as clothes on skin, warmth of sun etc. Press any key to move on to the next image.

See chapter 3 for more practical tips here.

4. FLASH CARDS

Flash cards are available in hands, feet, shoulders, backs and necks. Each set of flash cards consists of 48 images (24 images mirrored to equal a total of 48) that have been photographed with no interfering, contextual elements – for this reason we call them 'vanilla'. The images are generic and cover a range of positions and movements. Some will be easier than others, some are quite tricky. The images will be harder if they are sideways or upside-down. With each set of flash cards comes a booklet with some basic instructions and a few ideas about how to get the most out of your brain training exercises.

Hands, Feet and Shoulders

The question you should be asking here is 'Is this a left or right hand?' (foot or shoulder)

Backs and Necks

For implicit motor imagery tests with images of backs and necks, you should be asking: 'is this person turning to the left or right?'

4.1 PRACTICAL TIPS FOR USE

There are lots of popular games you can use to help with brain training exercises here – the distraction of fun being an additional benefit. These ideas can be easily modified for whichever set of cards you are using. Monitor your progress over time by recording your results on the work pages in the instructions booklet.

C 5

141

The Graded Motor Imagery toolbox
www.noigroup.com

GMI
hand
book

To add challenge and vary the context for a richer training exercise, you could take the cards from the comfort of your home to use in the park, your work place or the place where your injury happened. But gradually build up to this, don't throw yourself in the 'deep end'. You can use this technique of varying the environment, or context, or even adding distraction such as music for any of the suggested games. For example, sort the cards into two separate 'lefts' and 'rights' piles to a slow song and build up to a faster, boppier, or heavier song once you're feeling more comfortable. Using peaceful, your favourite or your least favourite music at different times is a simple means of adding emotional context to your exercises.

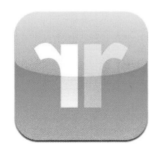

Figure 5.14
Recognise App icon

5. RECOGNISE APP

Here is a very accessible left/right discrimination retraining tool. Having the Recognise App (Figure 5.14) gives you motor imagery exercises at your fingertips on your phone – it's a bit like having a big and fancy set of flash cards in your pocket which gives you basic results in accuracy and response time (Recognise is far more complex). If you have a smart phone and access to the iTunes App store, it's a cheap, easy download so you can start using it straight away. Key features of the Recognise App are:

- You have the choice of vanilla, context and abstract tests

- Speed and accuracy results are recorded

- You can view your previous test results and your results as an average of all tests

- You have the option to entirely clear your results

- Each App is for a particular body part, (eg feet, hands, necks) – choose the one which suits you best

- You can take tests of between 2 to 50 images at once

- You have the flexibility to set the time displayed for each image

- There is no expiry date for Apps

6. OTHER USEFUL GMI TOOLS

6.1 MIRRORS, MAGAZINES, SEARCH ENGINES AND PHOTOS

Becoming resourceful and creative is an important part of GMI. Tim discusses the use of mirrors and magazines and other means of easily accessible brain training exercises in his chapter (chapter 3, 4.2.2). Why not try running a Google search for 'hand' images? Take a look through old family photo albums or jump on Facebook to dig up some past memories. You might want to take your own photos with a friend, tailored to suit your ideal exercises. Use these photos in Recognise or print them out to make your own flash cards.

6.2 CONTACT US

You might have been reading about 'out of the shadows learning' in David's chapter. We're really interested to hear about any experiences you've had – good or bad – using Recognise or any of the GMI tools. Your feedback helps to fashion and guide our ideas and contributes to the future of GMI tools.

In the header or footer of the Noigroup website (including Recognise) there is always a 'contact us' link. Go here to get in touch and share your thoughts, experiences, predictions or interesting results – we'd love to hear.

7. SUMMARY

We've come a long way from the ollies and manuals (maybe you even tried some yourself!) and hopefully the metaphor is now clear. We have designed Recognise, the Apps and flash cards using evidence from robust research, anecdotes and a dash of creativity to make these tools accessible and effective. In difficult times it will be useful to work alongside your clinician to help you persevere and maintain momentum in your graded approach to good health. Continue to problem-solve and brain-train at home and with your family so everyone understands the process. GMI hands you a wonderful opportunity to conquer your pain through patience, persistence, courage and commitment. It is a real modern treat – thanks to all the new things we now know from those hard at work at home, in the clinic and researching in the neuroscience world.

NOTES

INDEX

Noigroup Publications | 19 North Street Adelaide, South Australia 5000
+61 (0)8 8211 6388 | info@noigroup.com | www.noigroup.com
www.gradedmotorimagery.com | www.noigroup.com/recognise

GMI Resources

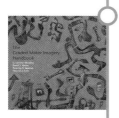

Graded Motor Imagery Handbook

Written by the principal researchers and educators of the GMI concept, this book will guide you through the science behind and the process of GMI. Graded motor imagery offers a novel three stage synaptic exercise process for neuropathic pain involving left/right discrimination, imagined movements and mirror therapy. With patience, persistence and often lots of hard work, GMI gives new hope for treatment outcomes.
The handbook is suitable for both patients and clinicians.

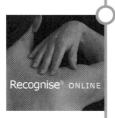

Recognise™

Even simple exercises may cause pain if your brain can't recognise whether you are using your left or right side. This can be tested easily and quickly using the Recognise programme. This novel evidence-based programme can provide valuable help in the management of many chronic pain states.

Flash Cards | These cards complement Recognise™ online and can be used for left/right discrimination or imagined movement excercises as part of the GMI process.

Online | A measurable, progressive self-management tool for patients. Test results can be collected and analysed. www.noigroup.com/recognise

App | The new Recognise™ App means you can quickly exercise your synapses on your smart phone or tablet wherever you are.

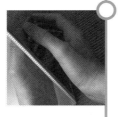

Mirror Box

Mirrors may be used to gain relief and better movement for a variety of pain and disability states, especially those involving the hands and feet. In particular, mirror therapy may be appropriate for problems such as complex regional pain syndrome, phantom limb pain, arthritis, stroke and focal dystonia. English / German / Italian / Portuguese

Explain Pain Resources

Explain Pain

Explain Pain and the philosophy and research behind it have become a huge influence on pain management across the English speaking world since its release in 2003. Still a ground-breaking concept in its content and presentation, this book aims to demystify the process of understanding and managing pain. It brings the body to life in a way that makes an interesting read for therapists and pain sufferers alike. Now available in five languages.

Explain Pain poster set

Select concepts from *Explain Pain* designed to encourage empowerment, helping pain sufferers to make informed choices and guide them to recovery: 'Take Control', 'Pacing Activity', 'Thought Viruses' and 'The Road to Recovery'. Use for a pain peer group setting, treatment room or waiting room wall.

Explain Pain audio

Combine reading with listening to make the most of the ground-breaking work of *Explain Pain* – Moseley and Butler talk you through. With over three hours of listening time on the CDs, reading is easier and retaining the knowledge more effective.

Painful Yarns

Written by clinical neuroscientist and co-author of *Explain Pain*, Lorimer Moseley, this book is an entertaining and informative way to understand modern pain biology. Described by critics as 'a gem' and by clinicians as 'entertaining and educative', the stories are backed by metaphors to pain biology. The level of the pain education is appropriate for patients and professionals, the entertainment is good for everyone.

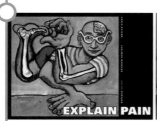
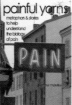

Neurodynamics Resources

Neurodynamic Techniques DVD & Handbook

NOIs international group of faculties presents the definitive manual of neurodynamic techniques for everyday clinical use. This DVD and Handbook will help with the assessment and management of physical health and sensitivity issues related to peripheral and central nervous system based pain presentations. Edited by Butler, DS.

The Sensitive Nervous System

This text calls for skilled combined physical and educational contributions to the management of acute and chronic pain states. It offers a 'big picture' approach using best evidence from basic sciences and outcomes data, with plenty of space for individual clinical expertise and wisdom. Butler, DS.

Red Wedge

Our wedge is light, strong and allows very localised active and passive mobilisation of joint and neural tissue in the thoracic spine. These techniques are demonstrated in the *Neurodynamic Techniques DVD and Handbook* and on NOI courses.

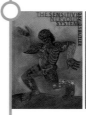
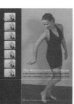
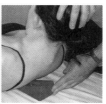

Noigroup Publications
19 North Street Adelaide, South Australia 5000
+61 (0)8 8211 6388 | info@noigroup.com | www.noigroup.com
www.gradedmotorimagery.com | www.noigroup.com/recognise